RECOVERY UNDERCOVER®

david emm

First published in 2001 by Red Rock Publishing, 1647-F Fellows, McMinnville, Or. 97128.

ISBN: 0-75964-230-3

This book is printed on acid free paper.

1stBooks – rev. 05/16/01

This book is dedicated to the memory of Mary Minton, a true inspiration to all who had the privilege to know her.

ACKNOWLEDGEMENTS

This author wishes to thank these people for their contributions: George Minton for his great help with storyline and review, Jan H. for her wonderful insight, Janalee Minton and Kathy Seery for their 'attaboys', León Flint for her much needed critique and most of all my wife Sam for her constant help with the daily process of keeping my writing honest.

A NOTE TO READERS

Although this is a story of good cops and bad guys, laced with a divinely appointed love affair; it is also a story about sober alcoholics, those special people who trudge the road of happy destiny, one day at a time. This book is dedicated to the millions of men and women, who once lived an existence of incomprehensible demoralization and have found their way back to a productive life. Every day, somewhere, recovery begins when one alcoholic talks to another, sharing his experience, strength and hope. Please note that the author's perception of the program of Alcoholics Anonymous is only an opinion. Some members may disagree with any part of AA as it has been represented it in this book this is a work of fiction. All the characters and events in this book are fictional. Any similarities to any persons, places or events are purely coincidental.

The following short list of definitions was included in the front of the book so that "normies" will not be left behind when two alcoholics are talking their special type of lingo:

BIG BOOK-The text titled Alcoholics Anonymous, first published in 1939. The original basis for the program called AA is contained in the first 164 pages, the remainder of the book contains personal stories of the members.

ANONYMITY-The AA tradition that keeps members from promoting their ego while at the same time protects those who could be harmed if their alcoholism were commonly known.

SPONSOR-A personal guide through the twelve steps of Alcoholics Anonymous.

MEETING-Two or more drunks getting together to discuss their experience, strength and hope.

GROUP-A loosely orchestrated group of alcoholics that meet regularly and are sanctioned by the national General Service Organization.

CLUB or CLUB HOUSE-A meeting place operated for the purpose of having AA and /or NA meetings. A club is totally separate from AA.

PROGRAM-The sober lifestyle that AA members endeavor to practice which includes working the steps, going to meetings, working with a sponsor and carrying the message to those who still suffer.

SOBRIETY-The total abstinence of alcohol (and/or drugs) in your life.

THE GRAPEVINE-The AA periodical.

BILL W.-Bill Wilson, the founder of AA.

DR. BOB-The other founding member of AA

ALCOHOLIC-A person who admits that he is powerless over alcohol.

DRUNK-Someone who may or may not have admitted that they are powerless over alcohol, but does indeed have a problem.

ALANON-A person who lives with the destruction of a practicing alcoholic, and the joyful confusion of a sober alcoholic.

INVENTORY-Personal moral list of transgressions and character defects.

OLD TIMER-Anyone with more sobriety than you.

HOW IT WORKS-From chapter five of the Big Book, the first few paragraphs.

HIGHER POWER-Your personal concept of a power greater than yourself.

HALT-Hungry, Angry, Lonely, Tired. Four of the triggers that can set an alcoholic to drinking.

THE 12 AND 12-Sometimes called the 12 by 12. The second most read book by people in the program. It contains the long versions of the twelve steps and the twelve traditions.

SOBRIETY DATE-The first day after the last drink.

AA COIN-A medallion that marks a length of sobriety such as one month, six months, one year or eleven years, ect.. Also called a chit, chip, or medal.

NORMIE-A normal person who does not have a problem with drugs or alcohol.

THE STEPS-See the twelve steps, code of principles and actions that can keep an alcoholic sober.

TRADITIONS- A set of twelve guidelines that has allowed AA to function world wide since 1946 with unity of purpose and only the loosest form of leadership.

THE PROMISES-From the Big Book pages eighty three and eighty four. The list of things sure to happen if you followed the twelve steps.

TABLE OF CONTENTS

Chapter 1: Larry.. page 1

Chapter 2: Conversations... page 11

Chapter 3: El Paso .... page 19

Chapter 4: Jackie... page 35

Chapter 5: The German .... page 42

Chapter 6: Mexico .... page 51

Chapter 7: Ruidoso .... page 69

Chapter 8 : The Italian .... page 78

Chapter 9: Serenity In The E R.. page 90

Chapter 10: Chihuahua .... page 104

Chapter 11: Dinner Guests.. page 119

Chapter 12: Truth, Lies And Consequences .... page 127

Chapter 13: Gunfight At The Hacienda... page 135

Chapter 14: Run For The Boarder .... page 146

Chapter 15: Hide And Seek .... page 161

Chapter 16: Lost And Found .... page 173

Chapter 17: New Beginnings .... page 187

Epilog... page 203

CHAPTER 1: LARRY

He leaned against the bathroom sink, staring at the face in the mirror. It was supposed to be his face, but he didn't recognize it. The face in the mirror was hard with deep creases and sunken eyes. His normally almond colored smooth skin was pale and blotchy. Reaching out, he touched the mirror, expecting to feel the pain that this face held. The mirror just felt cold and hard. Looking down at his wrist, he expected to see his gold watch; the one his wife had given him on their fifth anniversary. The expensive timepiece was gone, left behind in a Denver pawn shop. He could see the alarm clock by the bed. It was four in the morning. He turned back to the mirror and asked it, "who is this guy, and where is Larry?" It was the first time in over six months that Larry had really looked hard into a mirror. It was all over now, but he couldn't let it go. It was the hardest assignment he had ever been on, a deep cover operation for a joint drug enforcement task force. He had returned home to Albuquerque on an evening flight from Denver and came home to a hot, stuffy empty house. The only items she had left him, were the bedroom set, his personal stuff and the coffee brewer. She never drank coffee. He had drained the bottle of Baccardi from his suitcase and had fallen exhausted on the bed. Now, the face in the mirror haunted him with sallow cheeks, dead eyes complete with a road map of veins, and a scar that he couldn't connect to any memories above his eye. She had also left the bathroom scales behind, probably by mistake, because she watched her weight carefully. Stepping up, he learned that he weighed a mere one-hundred forty-one pounds. The last time he had been in this room he had weighed one sixty-eight. "Oh well, the booze must be good for my figure", he mumbled. "Who's voice is that!" He snapped at the face in the mirror. "Look pal, if you see Larry, send him back, cause I'm home now and I don't want to see you're ugly mug!" The face grinned an evil alcoholic grin, causing him to look away. Larry rummaged through his shaving bag and came up with one of those little booze bottles that you get on planes. He downed the contents and fell back on the bed, hoping for it to take effect. It wasn't enough booze to do any good. There were small insect-like creatures in day-glow colors crawling on the ceiling. They were laughing at him, they always laughed when he was short on booze. His whole body was dripping with sweat and he could feel his body shaking, but a part of his mind just thought it was someone else.

As he lay there, curled up in a fetal position, unable to let go of the fear, Larry tried to go over the past few months in his mind. His memories were patchy, at best. His daily life, running with Bumper Blue's gang of misfits, was sheer terror. Drug traffickers, that would kill at the blink of an eye and lived only by the code of who ever drinks or drugs the most wins. It was the most fear Larry had ever known. Other cops called what he did 'courageous', but he didn't feel courageous, just fearful. Everything he interacted with came with a fist full of fear. He couldn't sleep because it made him feel vulnerable. He felt he had to make some of the hardest of choices and pretend that it was normal behavior for him. Proclaiming that drugs are for light weights, he had showed them all how a real man could drink. After all, a cop wasn't supposed to do drugs, and he definitely had to do something to run with that wild bunch. He had seen Bumper kill a guy for hesitating on a line of coke. Larry was too scared to hesitate. He did what he had to do, then made them believe that he preferred the booze. It was an easy sell because, he really did like the booze. No harm in that, lots of cops drank hard. The booze could take the edge off the iceberg of fear. And in the end, he had got his man. Bumper Blue was in jail.

Sally his wife, no, ex-wife, had served him with divorce papers the day before he had left. She said it was over. She couldn't take the drinking and long periods of work related separation. Claimed that he was a different person every time he came home and that "all he ever did was drink and sulk." There was no use in trying to defend himself. He just accepted his fate, knowing that he had committed many indiscretions on his marriage while under cover. She would never understand. Larry certainly didn't look at himself as a bad man, the bad behavior could be justified Sometimes the booze gets it's own way. After all, love or not, she was in the way of his drinking. And he had to drink to survive, didn't he?

Sometime later, maybe the next day, Larry walked down to the market and pushed back a cart with a case of Baccardi light rum, three cases of silver bullets (Coors light beer) and a bag of chips. He told the cashier that he was throwing a party. The girl had her suspicions, but sold him the booze anyway.

Sometime later, maybe a few days, they found him in the back yard of his adobe style house where Sally had left an old rusty metal lawn chair. His feet were on the empty Baccardi box and his blue jeans were soiled from the inside. He was sitting in a puddle of urine and spilled rum. His eyes were rolled back into their sockets. The paramedics couldn't wake him up. The bag of chips lay unopened on the ground among the empty beer cans and Baccardi bottles.

Sometime later, maybe days or maybe a week, these two guys, with shinning faces were talking to Larry in the hospital. They said they were Joe and Bob, and they were going to help Larry with his problem. He thought maybe they could get him a drink. They said they had found a way out of the alcoholic haze that had ruined their lives, and they just wanted to share that with him. Larry felt awful. He was sad, remorseful, and depressed. His liver and his stomach both ached. But these guys had kind of an honest glow about them, and when they talked, they had shared feelings that Larry felt. They seemed to understand where he was coming from. He decided to listen but it was a hard thing to do at first. Joe and Bob didn't care, they said they were from AA and they would just keep coming back They were there when he was puking, and when he was screaming at everybody, and when he broke down and cried. One rainy morning they took turns holding him while he sobbed uncontrollably for several hours. In the end, Larry found a beginning.

SEVERAL MONTHS LATER

The room had its own ambiance. Not a big room, however, it had several banquet tables pushed together, making one larger center table with about twenty folding chairs around it; another thirty or so seats of various discarded styles lined the paneled walls. A short counter held an ancient restaurant style coffee warmer, cups and condiments. The aroma of fresh hot coffee mixed freely in the air with the pungent odor of nicotine left by hundreds of nervous smokers. On one wall a pull down shade displayed the 'Twelve Steps'. Ambitious persons, long forgotten, had printed signs with catchy slogans and tacked them close to the stained ceiling. Larry liked this room. Nothing here was pretentious, no complicated games to figure out. At home here, he felt none of the repressive tension that was normal to his occupation. If he was careful, speaking mostly in general terms, he could be himself in this room more than anywhere else. Outside was dangerous territory, where being guarded with his actions and speech had become second nature. Here in this room, it was just the fellowship of Alcoholics Anonymous, straight forward and simple.

His training as an undercover operative had taught him to always keep track of the people around him. It had become a compulsion for Larry to be aware that twenty two members had shown up for today's meeting. His skillful habit of instantly memorizing everyone's size, attire and attitude, never shut down. All of them where regulars today except for a smallish guy in a chair, sitting by the back door. Larry guessed he was a newcomer, probably sentenced by some well intentioned judge after being charged with drunk driving. The man looked so uncomfortable. Even with dark glasses, this guy had that scared defensive attitude, that out in the world could mean unpredictability and trouble. In this room, he was just one more suffering alcoholic that had yet to learn of the patience, love and forgiveness of these people. Larry made a mental note to talk to him after the meeting. After all, the Big Book says that you must help others to help yourself, and talking to newcomers was a good way to give back to the program. It was just a few months ago that Larry had been a newcomer, scared, angry, and uncertain of what to expect.

As for his own appearance, Larry was deliberately forgettable. Five foot nine inches tall, mid-thirties, slightly balding with a businessman's haircut and a nicely trimmed beard. For this part of his life, he wore silver wire-rimmed glasses that were just clear glass but helped him blend in. Larry didn't have an overtly muscular body, but, he was in shape from a daily five mile run along the Rio Grande river. He usually dressed 'Texas' style, in blue jeans, cowboy boots and a solid-colored button-down shirt. His heritage was a mixture of Irish and

Choctaw Indian, giving him an ethnic look of dark hair and light brown skin. Although, he was originally from Oklahoma City, he fit right into New Mexico's various mixtures of Indians, Latin Americans and Italians. Pure white Anglo Saxons are a minority in Albuquerque.

The sharp sound of knuckles rapping on the table instantly caught Larry's attention. An 'old timer', a veteran of thousands of meetings during his many years of sobriety, was opening the meeting. No matter how serene he tried to be, loud noises always seem to set off his internal alarm systems. No threat here, just time for the meeting.

"My name is Bob, and I'm an alcoholic," Started Bob. Amid a chorus of "Hi Bobs", he continued, "welcome to the noon meeting of Alcoholics Anonymous here at the High Plateau Club. We are self supporting, not allied with any denomination or sect, there are no dues or fees. This is an open meeting, Anyone may attend an open meeting. Let me remind you that anonymity is the foundation of our traditions. Who you see here and what you hear here, stays here. Please join me in a moment of silence followed by the serenity prayer."

"GOD GRANT ME THE SERENITY TO ACCEPT THE THINGS I CANNOT CHANGE, THE COURAGE TO CHANGE THE THINGS I CAN AND THE WISDOM TO KNOW THE DIFFERENCE. I'll now ask Suzie G. to read how it works from the Big Book."

As Suzie G., a blonde air head type, read the passage, Larry's attention wandered. He had managed to make two-hundred and twenty-four meetings in the last nine months of sobriety. He had heard the opening procedure enough times to have it all memorized. Bob was his sponsor, the person who guided Larry through the 'Twelve Steps' of Alcoholics Anonymous, he was a thin man, about sixty-five with serious eyes and fingers stained yellow from a lifetime of smoking.

Bob had been one of the first AA people to make contact with Larry. He had responded to a call from a friend of Larry's. Larry had been put on administrative leave after his last undercover assignment. That assignment had left Larry in bad shape from trying to fit in with a drug dealer's crowd. When Bob came to Larry's house, it was Bob who found Larry passed out, in the back yard, near death. Bob called the paramedics, cleaned him up and saw that Larry was taken to a detoxification center at a hospital, and then AA. It was Bob who helped Larry work through AA's 'Twelve Steps' the first time. Larry owed Bob everything, including his life.

Suzie G. finished 'How It Works' and Bob started Joe reading the 'Twelve Traditions'. Larry's mind shifted again. His eyes fell on Jackie, a nurse. As usual, she wore her crisp white uniform. Larry had heard her say she worked swing shift at University Hospital. His sponsor had warned him to stay away from AA women for at least a year and a half. Larry never understood what time had to do with emotions. But he was serious about his new found way of life and usually did what was suggested. Still, Jackie's demeanor haunted him. An attractive woman in her thirties of medium height, dark shoulder length hair, unusual green eyes and that "well scrubbed" professional look that came from years as an RN. Her heart shaped face was smooth and unusually pale for the desert country. Obviously, she stayed out of the sun a lot, just a few "wisdom" lines around the eyes. When he was a regular patrol cop, he had dealt with her type for years. Most of the nurses he found serious, but with a sense of humor. He had dated a number of RNs before marrying his ex-wife Sally, who was a dentist. But this one was different. Maybe it was this room that made her different. In this room people with good sobriety seem to have an honesty that is rare in society today. And after nine months of listening to Jackie's problems, opinions and feelings he felt a kin-ship to her. He did ask her out for coffee last week, only to be shut down abruptly. She said, "not to take it personally, but she just didn't see people in the program."

"For today's topic, let's talk about honesty", Larry heard Bob say, "For me, honesty is a tough subject. Maybe it is for some of you, too. One thing I've learned, in my nineteen years in this program, is that my concept of honesty changes as I grow in sobriety."

As Bob continued with his dry rhetoric, Larry remembered some of the ideas about honesty that Bob had helped him discover over the past few months. A lot of it had to do with the past. Bob said, "try and be as honest as you can everyday and don't worry about how honest you were yesterday." That was a big help for a while, then he had to do a 'Fourth Step', kind of a moral inventory of yourself and your past deeds. Honesty hits hard when you try to face both the past and the real you at the same time. Again, Bob's wisdom came to help. "Do your honest best, try not to cheat in your writings but don't worry about it. The only person doing any punishing, is you." After Larry had poured his heart into the 'Fourth Step', writing everything down that he could think of at the time, Bob made him do a 'Fifth Step', and a greater honesty came into play. In the 'Fifth Step', you have to share your moral inventory with God and another human being, in this case, it was Bob. It was just the first of several 'Fourth and Fifth Steps' that Larry and Bob did together over the last few months, each time using the process to clear away a little more wreckage of the past.

"Yeah, honesty must be really hard for a car salesman like you, Bob."

Larry heard Joe's good-natured jab at Bob. As everyone laughed at Joe's remarks and Bob mumbled something about Joe blowing his anonymity, the first word that came to Larry's mind was 'ouch'. Because Bob was his sponsor, it was hard not to take it personal when Bob spoke of some things. "How does someone who's whole life is built on lies and deceit become honest? ", Larry had asked him. It took six months for Bob to cut through Larry's tough exterior and discover the truth about Larry's complex life. The breakthrough happened while the two of them were having a 'Fourth Step' discussion, sitting on a rock by the Rio Grande river. Larry's sudden out burst and tears didn't shock Bob, he had seen it all during his long term sobriety. Bob had a lot of respect for Larry and empathy for his plight, but remained the tough sponsor because he knew eventually Larry would need every ounce of wisdom this program could offer, just to save his own life. Bob knew you couldn't save all of the suffering alcoholics and Larry might have a lot of suffering yet to do.

"The deception of others is nearly always rooted in the deception of ourselves", Larry heard Bob say. He now knew, that quote, was true about himself. He had deceived himself right up until they carried him out of the back yard. The booze had cost him everything, even his little girl, Jennifer. Just now he was learning what it meant to be honest and accept his own responsibility for it.

Larry's mind drifted back to Jackie. She was always a little aloof. Probably damaged goods, as some men would put it. Larry knew that sometimes people get hurt so deep in life that they can never recover enough to accept another loving relationship. What a waste that would be for Jackie. He thought she was so attractive and had so much to offer. Of course, it could be that she just didn't like him. Still, the honesty and purity of her AA program was captivating. She seemed so focused when she talked at the meetings. "Maybe someday, I'll be on her level of sobriety and then she will accept me enough to at least have that coffee.", he thought. As his daydream came back to reality, Larry realized Bob was calling on him to share.

"I'm Larry, alcoholic," he heard himself say. "Honesty is a bad subject for me, I probably need to listen more than I need to talk, but I hope someday I can understand what I really need to know about it. I still get confused with the different and shifting kinds of honesty you all talk about. The most honest I can be today, is to grab my butt with both hands and jump with both feet into this program, hoping for the best. At my stage of sobriety I feel like I don't know anything for sure. My sponsor says, "more will be revealed", so here I am. Thanks for letting me share."

That sounded stupid, Larry thought, contrite and pre-planned, like a good little AA parrot. She'll never think I've got a decent program that way. This brought an immediate mental reprimand to Larry's mind.

Not only was he taking Jackie's inventory, he was unfairly projecting his desires onto her. Larry had had enough sessions with Bob to know how wrong it was to think that way. "Resentments often come from expectations", Bob would say. Larry shook his head absently. Why did he have all these issues with Jackie when he didn't even know the lady? One of sobriety's puzzles, he guessed. More will be revealed.

"Hi everybody, my name is Albina and I'm you're token Al-anon for this meeting," Albino chuckled. "By the good grace of God and the help you and others like you have given me, I've been able to hold on to my practicing husband and what's left of my sanity. I'm new here so I'll let you know......"

Late fifties, with a tanned and well lined face, Albina looked the part of a worried wife who used gardening as a safety valve. Her slight build and hunched shoulders gave her the appearance of a victim. But Larry knew in his heart, that after all those years as a victim, she was now a hero. In all those years as a patrolman, domestic abuse calls were the most common. He remembered Albina from the old days. Arresting her husband on payday too many times to count. Sometimes she wore his violence on her face, but like many women, she had always refused to press charges the next day. Now she sat in this meeting having learned how to forgive the man who used to beat her. Standing by him in his sobriety as she had always done, but standing up for herself, also. Getting help for herself while her husband was getting help with his own AA program. Alcohol makes victims out of many family members and lots of them feel they have to lie to cover up the abuse and shame. Larry wondered if she recognized him.

"Thank you all for your help and understanding, I used think all drunks should be taken out and shot like crippled horses. Now, I know there is a way to live with this disease. Thanks for letting me share." Albina got up and started pouring coffee for everyone.

Larry smiled and nodded in her direction with admiration. He hoped the best for her and her man. "Hero's come in all sizes in the AA program", he thought. Bob called on Dave.

"My name is David and I'm an alcoholic. I really don't......"

Larry found himself wishing Jackie would get called on so he could here her voice and have a reason to look her way. He looked back at her anyway. She was looking at him and they locked eyes for a few seconds. He flushed and she glanced away.

Bob said, "We still have time for a couple of people to share before the clock runs out. Does anyone want to volunteer?"

"Yes. Jackie-alcoholic here," she said quickly. "I try to be honest too, but sometimes being honest isn't much fun. It can get you into trouble by being too direct or by saying more than a person needs to hear. Does this happen to you guys too? Like when someone asks something of you and you answer with a pat answer before you get a chance to think through the consequences of what you are saying. It is real easy to hurt other people without knowing it because you are too, "in their face", with your honesty. I must like the taste of shoe leather, because I stick my foot in my mouth several times a day. My dear sponsor tells me that this is why we have the 'Ninth and Tenth Steps', so that we can make amends to those people we may hurt even if we didn't mean too. The Big Book says, on page seventy, "If we are sorry for what we have done, and have the honest desire to let God take us to better things, we believe we will be forgiven

7

and will have learned our lesson. If we are not sorry and our conduct continues to harm others, we are quite sure to drink." The folks who wrote the book were talking about the damage their drinking had done, but I think it is a good principal to put in my everyday life because it's not just about being sober. For me, it's also about being a better person tomorrow than I feel I am today. Thanks Bob for letting me share."

Larry felt himself reaching out mentally to Jackie. Letting her words wrap him up in safety and security. He couldn't help himself, everything she said or did seemed perfect to him. Oh, to be close to a woman like that. Not very likely, though, considering his occupation and failed marriage.

"Before we close I would like to acknowledge the young man in the back. I don't think we've met, but you are welcome here. Would you like to tell us your first name so we can say a proper hello to you?"

Everyone in the room turned a friendly face to the newcomer. Larry refocused his attention. He had learned that newcomers are important to sobriety. He had been a newcomer not so long ago.

"It's Darin. The judge said I had to come here everyday for a month because it was my second DUI. I thought he was being stupid, but y'all are all-right. Maybe I do have some sort of problem. At least I know that I can't stop drinking for very long. I tried to keep away from the booze for a week last month. And y"all are talking "bout being honest today so I gotta say, I didn't make it. I expected to get a test here today 'cause the judge said y"all had a test to see if I had a problem with drinkin'. When do I have to take it? Guess that's all I have to say."

"I think you just passed it," Said Joe.

Bob joined in, "We are glad you are here, Darin, if you think you might have a problem, you probably do, and if you have a desire to stop drinking, then you are in the right place. If you stick around after the meeting, some of us would like to talk to you and maybe give you some phone numbers to call if you want our help. Please keep coming back. If for no other reason than that the judge says so."

"Shall we close in the usual manner?," Bob stated, "Katherine, would you like to lead us in The Lord's Prayer?" Everyone stood and held hands.

Katherine paused and started, "Our Father, who........................"

Larry peeked at Jackie during the prayer. Her head was back, exposing her exquisite long neck, her eyes were closed, brown hair falling on her shoulders. Her face beamed like an angel as she recited. Larry closed his eyes, feeling more doubt about his self-worth, but remembering how perfect she looked.

After the meeting Larry helped clean up a little and was the third person to talk to Darin. He discovered Darin was from west Texas, and a welder. He had moved to Albuquerque when the oil-field work slowed down. Now he welded for a defense contractor, who was on contract for Sandia Labs. Larry knew how touchy defense jobs were. If Darin had another DUI, he would be out of a job.

Jackie was talking to Katherine, her sponsor. It looked like a serious conversation. Katherine left in a hurry, before Larry finished talking to Darin. Jackie stayed behind puttering with the coffee cups. Very unusual. Katherine and Jackie normally left together because they both worked at the hospital. Larry gave Darin his phone number and told him he would be glad to have coffee with him after a meeting sometime. Then he noticed that all others had gone except Jackie. Thinking Jackie might want to talk to Darin, Larry made his good bye and started to leave.

Jackie caught his arm in the parking lot and said, "Hey you, I just want to say I'm sorry for brushing you off last week. Just because you are in the program, doesn't mean you are an untouchable or something. We could have coffee before a meeting someday. As long as it's daylight and in public we can't get into too much trouble. How about tomorrow at the Sunshine Café, say, ten thirty?"

Larry was floored. He didn't know what to say except, "yeah, okay." As she drove off in her late model Toyota, he just stood there stunned. It occurred to him that he might be reliving his childhood or at least his high school years. He felt like such a teenager. His heart pounded, his knees were weak and he had forgotten to breath. Slowly a huge smile spread across his face like sweet honey on a hot biscuit. He had the urge to jump in the air and yell, but years of being an adult kept his feet on the ground.

Later that evening Jackie and Katherine were having their lunch on one of the hospital's outdoor patios, enjoying the summer evening. For August, the heat wasn't too bad this year. Summertime in the five thousand foot city could be unbearable at times, but for now, the warm fresh air was just what the two women craved after several air-conditioned hours in rooms filled with the scent of deliberate sanitation. Conversation between these good friends flowed easily like a babbling creek down a mountain side. Eventually they turned their attention to Jackie's fascination with Larry. Katherine's responsibility to help Jackie keep herself out of trouble, both as a sponsor and a friend, was tainted by her desire to see her friend shake herself out of her autonomous existence.

"I don't know, it's your call. I can only make a few suggestions."

"Yeah but, your 'suggestions' are full of AA experience and great Native American philosophy. I think I need all the help I can get on this one."

"Okay, forget the fact that this guy is only a few months sober. Why are you still so reluctant to get involved if you are so attracted to him?"

"I suppose it's based in fear. Like everything else I do."

"Oh don't go pitiful on me. Fear is a learned experience, not a character defect. It's okay to be afraid, especially for a new experience. You know your not exactly the date-queen of Albuquerque."

"We aren't going out on a date. We just agreed to have coffee in the morning."

"Is that what he thinks?"

"Well, that's what he first asked me, and I turned him down, but you know me, sometimes, I get tired of just work and AA."

Katherine fingered her beaded necklace. "Well then, what's the problem. You work hard and have a good program-you deserve a little recreation."

"That's part of the problem, in my heart, I want more than recreation. And then there's my past, and his newness to sobriety to add to the equation. I'm not sure that I'm wise enough to do all the right things to keep both of us sober."

"His sobriety isn't your responsibility. He has Bob for a sponsor, you know. He has help on his end and he is a big boy, too. Don't try to control everything. The 'Great Spirit' has that job. Do you want to know what my ancestors would say?"

"Is this another story about the rabbit and the hawk?"

"No, they'd say to follow 'Rule 62'. You know what that is, 'don't take yourself too seriously.'"

"Yeah but,....."

"No 'yeah buts' about it girl, just follow your feelings and let your higher power sort it out."

"I guess that I'm more scared than a teenager going to the prom. I think I can handle the coffee and conversation, but, I don't know what comes next. Is that fear or too much control?"

"Why don't you just call it adventure and enjoy yourself?"

"Okay, I guess I'm just an emotional wimp."

"No, you just need to get out more. We better get back to work. This fresh air might be habit forming."

CHAPTER 2: CONVERSATIONS

When Larry arrived at the Sunshine Café, the place was buzzing. It was a beautiful southwestern summer morning and the café in the college district was living up to it's name. The big plate glass windows and skylights let the sun stream down on the dozens of healthy green plants. Two weeks had passed and Larry was showing up for his fifth 'coffee date' with Jackie. He really looked forward to these all too brief times together. Getting to know her was probably the biggest pleasure he had known in sobriety, even if he often felt like the court jester in front of 'Her Royal Majesty'.

Jackie sat by a window looking deep into a cup of coffee. A pleasant look on her face. The sight of her made him gasp, for him, she was the best looking woman he knew. However, everything about her seemed a little different today. A little neater, a bit more put together and somehow more beautiful. The dark green pants suit was a perfect compliment to her green eyes and he noticed a very subdued make up job. Jackie rarely wore makeup, and usually wore jeans and T-shirts when not working. He wondered if she was going to attend a special event . As he neared the table, the pleasant fragrance of perfume overcame his senses, it was the first time that he noticed her using perfume. She didn't notice his approach and was startled by his greeting.

"They say all good answers can be found in a cup of hot coffee. Good morning. You're a nice sight to see in the morning." He said causing her to jump, then blush.

Jackie quickly regained her composure. "Oh, thanks. I'm glad you're here", she returned. "How are you this morning?"

"I'm fine. Did I disturb you concentration? You looked like you had a lot on your mind."

"I was just thinking about all the changes that I have gone through since I became a sober person. You are fairly new and may not understand what you are going to go through."

"What ever it is, I sure hope I'm up to it", quipped Larry, "sounds like pretty heavy thinking for a bright sunny morning like this."

Jackie stared at him pensively before answering. "Do you ever doubt your ability to stay sober? It's normal if you do, you know." She brushed her fingers through her soft hair and smiled.

"Well, I do have a desire to stay clean and sober, and I don't have a desire to drink, too often", Larry said in return, hoping she would focus on the desire and drop the third degree stuff. "Do you think I can make it? You know, I respect your opinion, you've got such a good program going."

"When you say clean and sober it usually means you've had experience with drugs. I don't remember you saying anything about drugs in the meetings", she said.

It was Larry's turn to be pensive. He thought carefully before answering. "I wasn't sure whether or not it was okay to talk about it at AA meetings, being that the subject is alcohol. Most of the street drugs, I've tried. Not too much problem with them though, most of the time I stayed with my rum, vodka, and beer where I was more comfortable. Not all at the same time of course. Does it bother you that I experimented a little?"

"No, in my book, it's no worse than alcohol. I am glad you realize that booze was your biggest concern. A lot of people try to blame the drugs for their drinking, but usually, they were drinking in excess when they started on the drugs. I believe the drinking is where you have to change your life. Fix that, and the rest will follow. Oh golly. I'm sorry to get on a soap box with you. I hardly know you and you aren't a newby with, nine months, is it?"

Jackie felt like a fool for spouting off like that too this nice man. She didn't come here to continue to step on him. Her intentions were far different this morning. She no longer struggled with why was she compelled to meet him like this. She just accepted that something was developing between them and she made the decision to just enjoy her interaction with Larry and see what happens. It was a brave decision for her.

"Wow you really are heavy this morning. No need to apologize to me. I'll treasure absolutely anything you tell me." What a teenage type of thing to say Larry thought as he felt the blood rush to his cheeks. Looking up at Jackie, he saw her face was flushed also.

"Look, I'm sorry if I embarrassed you Jackie. Can I be frank with you? Its just that I think you are terrific, and all of a sudden, I don't know how to act." As the words fell out of his mouth, he thought he heard his voice crack. "I know we aren't teenagers, but that is the best way to describe how I feel."

"Larry", Jackie started, "Have you heard about the thirteenth step, yet?"

Larry said that he heard it in a meeting once, then everyone laughed. His pulse quickened as he realized there might be a chance of advancing their relationship.

Jackie continued, "The thirteenth step is when a person of more sobriety, usually the opposite sex, uses that knowledge and experience to take advantage of someone with less sobriety. Sometimes it's financial, sometimes emotional, or, maybe even the person with more sobriety is a sexual predator. That is why all the old timers and sponsors say not to date program people for quite a while. It is a big responsibility to get your character defects intertwined with other 'alkies'. Even in the most innocent form, it opens the door to a lot of misunderstanding."

"Do you mean that you are going to 'Thirteenth Step' me?" He realized what he had just blurted out and tried to make it a joke by laughing unconvincingly. Jackie paused and went on in a serious tone.

"I think I must be more than a little attracted to you, and that really complicates my life and sobriety. The danger is that you are at a level of sobriety where I could, with my four years of sobriety, unscrew your head and leave you hurting enough to blow your program. Do you understand? How do you know that I'm not going to play a bunch of head games with you for my own sick pleasure and then dump you in an emotional gutter? The question you need to ask yourself is, 'is it worth it'?" It quickly occurred to her that he might think she was trying to push him away. She didn't realized that she had asked the question.

Larry was almost speechless, but managed a nod and a grunt of some sort. After an embarrassed pause, while she studied his face, a change came over him. He smiled and looked deep into her eyes.

"The answer is yes." His voice was low and even, leaving no question as to his intent. She could not shift her eyes from his gaze. She opened her mouth to say something, but nothing came out. She was a prisoner of the moment, caught by the inevitable truth. He continued, his self-assured male instincts trumping her four years of sobriety. At least for the instant.

"You know, I really do have feelings for you ...." He decided he was being overbearing as his mind suddenly dropped him back in reality. Although his soul screamed to profess undying love for her, his mind backed down. He looked down and away for a moment, then went on. "I think I understand what you are trying to say. Maybe we should set down a few ground rules. It appears that our friendship is about to change."

Jackie realized that she wasn't breathing. "Well," she said as she took a deep breath, "that's probably a good idea." Her senses were alive and vibrating. It took effort to keep the emotional distance that had become her habit. She took another deep breath and reached out and touched his hand on the table.

"Your quite a guy, Larry, let's start with no touchy-feely in or around AA meetings. We have to keep the sanctuary of the meetings sacred. Agreed?"

"I can see that."

"And we both need to work with our sponsors."

"Of course, that almost goes without saying."

"Larry, I like you and we have had some nice conversations about sobriety and my work, but I hardly know anything about you."

"I don't want it to sound like black mail, but if you'll have dinner with me tonight, I'll tell you what I can."

"You mean, like a real date?"

"Yeah, and I'll even throw in a movie, if it will help you say yes."

"Did you know it was my day off or just a guess?"

13

"I have my ways, we can talk about that later, over dinner."

"Okay, you've charmed me into dinner and a movie. How about seven o'clock?"

"Sounds good, I'll pick you up." He rose and lightly touched her face before leaving. It occurred to her that he hadn't asked for her address.

At seven o'clock sharp Larry was at Jackie's apartment door. She was ready, wearing a long blue denim skirt with a crisp white blouse accented by a turquoise 'squash blossom' necklace. He escorted her to the pearl white Cadillac that he had rented for the night. The broken down Ford he usually drove didn't seem right for what he hoped was a special night.

"Nice car," she said feeling the soft leather against her form. "I didn't know you had more than one car."

"I suppose I could pretend, but I gotta be honest. This is a rental, it just seemed more appropriate for our first date."

"Yes, a girl likes to be impressed. We'll pretend together. Have you picked out a great restaurant?"

"Uh huh, have you ever been to the 'High Financial Restaurant'?"

"No, where's it at?"

Larry chuckled. "It's the highest restaurant in Albuquerque, you'll see." He turned left from Candelaria onto Tramway Boulevard. Jackie watched the houses slip by until they reached the edge of the city. When the Cadillac turned back towards the Sandia Mountains, her face lit up with laughter.

"I get it! It must be the restaurant at the top of the tramway. I've heard of the place, but didn't know the name. Does this include a ride up the tram?" She was truly excited.

"Yep." Larry knew he had made the correct assumption-that Jackie had not been for a ride on Albuquerque's famous tramway.

"I am impressed!" She squeezed his hand.

They both stood up to have the optimal view for the ride up the mountain in the famous Sandia Peak Aerial Tramway. There were two other couples in the car built to hold about twenty, but nobody spoke much. All present were awed by the spectacular view during the 2.7 mile lift up the slope. The city, the Rio Grande river and desert reaching out beyond; it was beautiful in the summer evening.

Larry ordered prime rib for both of them and they settled into their salads and conversation.

"Okay, mystery man, your on. It's your turn to let someone know who you are and what you're about."

"What would you like to know? My full name is Larry Patrick Kelly, I'm thirty seven years old, divorced, father of one."

"Gee, that's a good start," she mocked him with a twinkle in her eye. "What kind of work do you do."

"I could tell you, but then I'd have to ruin the evening by killing you." He said in his best Sean Connery-James Bond accent. She laughed. "Actually, I'm on a sabbatical from work while I get my sobriety together."

Jackie sensed that she shouldn't push the subject. "Kelly sounds Irish, I would have thought you were of a Spanish heritage, or maybe Italian."

"Everyone thinks that. My mom was Choctaw Indian and my father was an Irish cop."

"Is that what you are, a cop of some sort?" It just slipped out and from the look on his face, she was sorry she had brought it up again.

He leaned forward across the table and spoke in a quiet voice. "Jackie, you'll probably get to know me better, but please don't pry about my work." He hesitated. "To answer your direct question, sort of, but I'm not allowed to talk about it. Just know that I make an honest living on the right side of the law."

"I'm sorry, I didn't mean to pry. With most people, it doesn't matter. If you need your privacy, it's your right. Please forgive me."

"No harm done, I don't mean to be mysterious, it's just the people that I work for require…"

"Okay, can you tell me about your ex-wife and child?" She tried to change the tone of the conversation.

"My wife's name was Sally, she was a professional woman, a dentist. Not much of a story there, you've heard some of it at meetings. She hated my job and I drank away our marriage. It's the usual alcoholic story." His face softened. "My girl's name is Jennifer. I miss here dearly. She was just a five year old bundle of love last time that I saw her. They live in northern California now. I don't know if, or when, I'll get to see her again. I need to be completely straightened out before I can make that request. I promised Sally that in the divorce. She said I could visit all I wanted with Jenny as long as I stayed sober."

"I bet Jennifer is a sweetheart. Was that Sally Kelly, the dentist with the office over on Juan Tabo Avenue? I have a friend who went to her."

"That's the one. How about you? I know that you're a nurse, at the hospital, right?"

"Yeppers, nurse Jackie, at your service. Oh, I work the trauma center on the swing shift. It's a good job. University Medical is a busy place."

"Yeah, I've been to the ER. Not much stand around time there."

"Right, most people don't know it but we take the worst patients from all over New Mexico and parts of Arizona and Colorado. They fly them in from everywhere it seems."

The two ate and talked over coffee until they were the last diners. The sun was disappearing behind the desert hills and the lights were twinkling on in the city below. They had the tram car to themselves for the trip down the mountain.

15

Sitting on the hard fiberglass bench, Larry put his arm protectively around Jackie's shoulder. The view was breathtaking at night, but Larry could only look at her. Neither spoke, each lost in thought about their new found relationship. At her door, she held him tight. He was a gentleman and didn't push himself on her.

"Larry, thanks for tonight." She whispered. "It's been a long time since I felt so happy and relaxed. I think we can have real feelings for each other, at least I'm pretty sure about me. But, I do think we need to go slow."

"No problem, 'Little Lady', it's my pleasure." He said in a bad John Wayne imitation. "I had a good time, too, and I know we have lot's of things to deal with. I guess it's hard not to be clinical about it when we sit around analyzing our lives every day."

She smiled and turned her face towards his. Her penetrating green eyes gave him goose bumps in the night air. Reaching up, she took his face in her warm hands. "Larry, I......" He leaned forward cautiously, and gently kissed her.

His beeper went off and the special moment clasped into the real world. It took him a few seconds to understand that the annoying sound came from his belt.

"Damn, it's me," he looked at the display. "Well, I've got to go make this call. Sorry, 'Little Lady', duty calls."

"You can come in and use my phone."

"Believe me, I'd like to, but, the rules are to use a payphone, so I've gotta go. Can we do this again someday."

"Yes, call me."

He hugged her again and left. She watched through her window as he pulled away. She felt warm and fuzzy, this man could be the best thing to happen to her in a long time.

The number on Larry's beeper was that of his boss, Captain Moffit. Larry knew the number well. Although he was on administrative leave, Larry still had court appearances and technical input to the case on Bumper Blue and the drug traffickers he worked so hard to bust. So, the Captain called him several times a month. When he returned the call, Captain Moffit requested a meeting at a park across the river in the suburb of Rio Rancho. After becoming a 'deep cover' agent, Larry never went into any police station unless he was in handcuffs. The thought of a clandestine meeting with his boss put an old feeling in Larry's stomach, like performing in a carnival high wire act without a net.

Larry arrived at the park at nine AM the next morning. He parked his nondescript Ford at the mini-mart across the street and circled the park on foot, knowing even the captain could make mistakes that could be fatal. Everything seemed normal except, Moffit's uncomfortable form, resting on a park bench, trying to eat a messy breakfast burrito from a street vendor. He was totally unaware of Larry's approach.

16

"You really should turn up that hearing aid when you are out in the open, sir.", Larry said from behind the bench. Moffit jumped up spilling picante sauce on his shirt.

"Damn it man," he answered, "why do you always do that to me? You know my left ear hasn't worked sense that grenade went off in that crack house last year."

Captain Moffit was a tall bulky, barrel-chested man in his late fifties, with a full head of white hair and that distinguished look of a television Mafia Don. Moffit was Larry's only remaining contact with the Albuquerque police force, and the go-between for Larry and the "Feds". Larry felt this was the man he worked for, but he was really on loan to what ever agency needed his services. Larry had worked for the Justice Department, DEA, FBI, ATF, IRS, INS, and Customs. His pay checks were direct deposited from a consulting firm in Boston. The job was always the same. Get the evidence and get out of harms way before the bust. It was always dangerous. Larry walked a fine line between terror and duty. Some assignments were easy and short, others were hard and long. The last one, had really taken a toll on Larry's life. He lost his wife, daughter and house-his grounding rod to normalcy. If it wasn't for Captain Moffit's recommendation, he would have lost his job, also. That might have been a good thing, only the future will tell. In the end, he came out of that assignment a drugged out drunk. Now if the prosecutors did their job right, it would all be worth it. He had helped take Bumper Blue, his real name was Warren Smith, off the streets. And Bumper was the worst kind of trafficker, dealer and murderer.

"What's up?", Larry queried.

"There's a little situation that Treasury needs some help with. Are you ready to go back to work?" Moffit began, "I know I promised you a year to get those monkeys off your back, but the bad guys don't even take Sundays off."

Larry felt his whole world slip away into the desert sun. Duty called and it was always important. He knew he wasn't ready to go back undercover. His knees went weak. His eyes watered. His heart raced. And his mouth said, "Yes, sir. Where am I off to this time."

"Probably El Paso to start," Moffit said with a mouth full of juicy ingredients. "It's come up that Bumper was involved in a counterfeiting group across the border. The scuttle-butt is, the cash is made in Mexico, brought in around El Paso and shipped here to Rio Rancho where several Mafioso types have retired. It's assumed, that they move it from here to both, the east and west coast for distribution."

"Don't we have enough on Bumper, Captain?"

"This ain't about Bumper. He was just transportation in this ring. The 'Feds' want the bigger fishes, as usual."

"What's my cover and when do I start?" Larry inquired. The old feeling of nervous energy was creeping in.

"You have already started. Take the silver minivan over there and go to El Paso. There is an identity package on the seat and the name of a Treasury Department undercover contact in El Paso." Moffit's eyes turned to stone, leaving no room for argument.

Larry almost said something in protest, but he knew by Captain Moffit's look that they were being watched. Probably the ''Feds'', they liked to play those games. He slid into the seat, turned the key and headed for Interstate Twenty-five.

A faint odor of expensive perfume told Larry that the mini van belonged to a woman. Enforcement agencies, especially the ''Feds'', used a lot of confiscated vehicles for their undercover work. Real cars for phony people was the way Larry thought about it.

El Paso was a long drive from Albuquerque and it gave him a lot of time to think. He was curious about the assignment and even more curious about how long it would take. Duty was not always fair. He was just starting to feel comfortable with his sobriety and it was a scary thought that he would be away from his support group for the first time since leaving the hospital. In the back of his mind, there was a small cloud of doubt. The doubt was about his ability to go back and do the same police work sober, that he used to do drunk. He still had his training and his experiences, but something was different. Maybe it was his willingness or maybe it was fear. It was hard to put his mental finger on it. He just hoped it would not interfere with the job at hand. Then there was the situation with Jackie. Finally off to a good start, and now an unexplainable absence. He was certain she would think he was some sort of "flake."

After stopping for gas at Socorro, an odd thing happened. As Larry pointed the silver van up the freeway ramp, he noticed a dead armadillo laying on it's back at the side of the road. Coming to a stop, he realized someone had propped a long neck beer bottle up in the animals paws, giving it the appearance of a drunk armadillo. It was hard not to take it as an omen and it upset him enough to get out and move the poor dead creature behind a bush. It may have been a funny joke to some, but it just disgusted Larry. After that, his mood had changed and he spent most of the trip mentally reviewing the skills that would keep him alive while under cover.

CHAPTER 3: EL PASO

Larry pulled into the City Center Motel in Las Cruces, New Mexico. About fifty miles short of El Paso, Texas. He needed someplace to review the case and his new undercover identity. A Mediterranean looking woman, with a ring in her nose, issued him the key to room 112. It was a typical mid-priced room, clean, but with worn bedding and scratched furniture. Not quite a dive yet. A sliding glass picture window on the back side, not only gave a great view of the San Andres mountains, but also provided an emergency escape route, although, Larry doubted the need to escape so early in an operation.

Spreading the contents of the envelope on the bed, he started the process. The envelope contained several papers with Department of the Treasury letter heads and two glossy photographs. Larry picked up a page titled "OVERVIEW", which explained the three objectives of the mission. The first priority is to find out the when, the where, and the who, concerning the next large shipment of counterfeit money into the USA. The second priority is the location and the status of the plates being used to make the money. And third is the location and security details of a man named Al Bennette, an exiled Mafia Boss, who was said to be in charge of this counterfeiting operation. The overview went on to define Larry's roll as that of a spy, not an enforcement tool. He was meant to infiltrate the organization, by the means provided, and bring out information only.

One photo was of a square faced, Earnest Borgnine looking guy about sixty-five years old, with a big cigar stuck in the corner of his mouth. The picture was taken on a raining day in Chicago as the man crossed the street near the CBS building. The man carried a most unpleasant expression. Larry knew Chicago, having done a month for the FBI in Chicago, bringing down a Mexican slave labor ring. He doubted that these two cases would have any of the same people involved. That was always a nasty possibility when you do a lot of undercover operations. A short dossier informed him of Bennette's long crime career with the Chicago mob as an enforcer, executioner and neighborhood boss. When the federal prosecutor made a move to shut down his operations and arrest him, the Mafia bosses arranged a smugglers flight to Mexico for him and his key people. Bennette had taken up residence somewhere south of El Paso.

The other photograph was a red headed man in a cheap suit, a typical bureaucratic law man. Too clean and polished to be much else. A successful business man would wear a better quality suit, and a good cop would at least have a food stain on his tie. A telephone number was written in felt tip pen on the front, and a dress code for Larry to be identified by, described on the back. An envelope was attached to the picture with a lime green, two inch button that said, "REAL COWBOYS DON'T LINE DANCE." The front of the envelope listed the basic details of Larry's cover identity. Inside were a passport, four credit cards, a video store card, Arizona drivers license, and a picture of a small brown dog in the arms of a pale woman. His new name is to be Tom Sullivan, nick named "Sully", from Phoenix, Arizona. Sully was a "made man" in the Las Vegas mob who had been moved to Phoenix to oversee illegal gambling joints and to act as a liaison to the new Native American casinos. The real Sully was in protective custody on a military base somewhere in Wyoming and was apparently cooperating.

Sully was described as a cowboy with a quick and unyielding temper. To Larry's amazement, Sully was a teetotaler and hated drugs. One of Larry's big fears was having to play the part of a drunk or drug user. In criminal circles, use and abuse were common. To not do the drug or take the drink could mean exposure and death. "Wow, my higher power is really at work here today!", he said out loud.

After carefully committing all the details to memory, Larry disconnected the smoke detector alarm in the room so he could burn the papers and photographs in the sink. Sitting back on the bed, he checked the weapons that had been left for him in the van. The big one was a ten shot Glock nine millimeter with two loaded clips and a shoulder holster. The small one was a five shot thirty-two caliber automatic with an ankle holster. The treasury guys must think this is dangerous to make sure he was armed, or maybe Sully was known to carry these guns. He made a mental note to stop at a sporting goods store before he left Las Cruces and buy new rounds for both units. When your life depends upon it, you don't leave such things to strangers. Guns made Larry nervous. Most of his missions did not require a gun. A tape recorder and a spy camera were usually his only armaments. "What would I tell my sponsor if I actually had to shoot someone?", he mused, "Bob would have a cow on that one."

Being about eight-thirty, Larry was hungry, so he walked across the parking lot to the restaurant. On the way he stopped at the pay phone to call his contact, but no-one answered. On the door of the restaurant banquet room was a sign displaying the familiar triangle within the circle that meant an AA meeting could be found there. Sitting in an empty booth, he debated about one last meeting before going underground. When he mentioned the sign to the waitress, she said an eight o'clock meeting was about over, but that he was welcome to carry his coffee back to the banquet room if he wanted. She was obviously in the program. He thanked her and just sat there not knowing what to do. Las Cruces was very close to El Paso and the risk of exposure was great. It wasn't fair for the universe to tempt him with something so good that could be so wrong for this operation. He decided to order a steak and apple pie instead of more sobriety.

As Larry was polishing off the apple pie, a tall cowboy approached the table. "Forgive me for intruding", the cowboy said, "my name is Trevor. Rose, the waitress, said you might be a friend of Bill W.'s Most folks just call me "T"."

Not wanting to draw attention to himself, Larry smiled and said, "Please, sit down. They call me Sully. Thanks for coming over. I was just too hungry to go to the meeting. You know, the HALT thing can really get me sometimes. Just sort of sneaks up on me." Larry tried to hold back his combination of relief and enthusiasm. Sully probably wasn't too friendly. He wished he knew if Tom Sullivan was in the AA program. Oddly enough, a lot of criminal types found AA in jail or prison. Even though they some how found justification to go on being a bad guy, they somehow found room for sobriety in their lives.

Trevor was six feet six, late fifties or early sixties; dressed in work jeans, boots, denim shirt, straw cowboy hat and a big rodeo prize buckle. When he smiled, his leathered face seemed to crack in a hundred places. He ordered coffee from Rose, who now wore a look of warm satisfaction. "Hey, do it any way you want," Trevor started, "no-one tells me how to run my program, and I can't tell anybody else, either. I travel a lot with the rodeo circuit, so I certainly know what it's like to be a stranger."

"Are you a rodeo performer?", Larry asked.

"No. Too old and busted up for that these days. I'm a professional rodeo judge, but mostly I go out on the circuit because I think my higher power wants me to be there when ever my friends have had enough of the drinking and parties," he answered.

"What was the topic of the meeting tonight?" Larry questioned, glad for the company, but wanting to keep the conversation away from himself.

"Tonight we were talking about amends. I don't suppose you've had to make any of those, have you Sully?" Trevor offered with a big smile and knowing twinkle in his eye. "I'll tell you, I've had to make some tuff ones. Us cowboys tend to get a little wild once the booze takes over our judgment. Know what I mean, Sully?"

Larry liked this big cowboy and was happy that he wanted to talk about his experiences instead of Larry's. "Yeah, I'll have to admit, there's been a few. Go ahead and tell me a few of yours. I could stand to hear that right now."

"Well, tonight I shared about a little incident that happened about nine years ago. Me and the bull riders were whooping it up pretty good over in San Angelo, Texas after the semi-finals. I was bragging about my Marine Corps days when this city cop decided we needed arresting. Being that there was four of us and one of him, he pulled his gun. Probably a rookie. Anyway, I did a little ju-jitsu move on him and took his gun away. Then, to let everyone know what a big man I thought I was, I stuck his badge in his mouth and his gun under his chin until a few more cops came to take me away. It was just me and a bottle of Jack Daniels having fun. Didn't mean no harm. The judge didn't see it that way and I did eighteen months. Ended my rodeo career and my drinking at the same time."

"The booze seems to take the things you love, don't it?" Larry added.

"Boy howdy, ain't it the truth," Trevor laughed, "last year I decided to make amends to that cop. I found him in Big Springs, still a policeman. What impressed the hell out of me, was that he remembered everything about that night. The time, date, the weather, what I was wearing, the case number and everything else. He said that his memory of that act, had terrorized him for years. He had actually wet himself, he was so scared. Also, he said he had lived in constant fear that someone else would get his gun and kill him. Not to mention the embarrassment when the other cops showed up. We talked for a couple of hours. I explained my AA life style and how I was trying to clear up my past. In the end he forgave me and wished me well, but he said he still wouldn't sleep any better. I guess, we can do a lot of damage out there when we get drunk."

Trevor's story really hit home with Larry. A cops nightmare. He wished he could tell him about some of his own scary experiences as a police officer. Instead he let Trevor ramble on about his drinking and rodeo friends, making the appropriate AA comments at the correct places. After an hour or so, he excused him self, shook hands and left.

Walking back across the parking lot, Larry realized that life was not the same for him while undercover. This would have to be his last covert assignment. It is just too dangerous to be thinking about, and reacting to, his sobriety when he should be watching his back. He stopped a second time at the pay phone hoping to make contact with the red headed treasury man; still no answer. After taking a few steps towards the room, he turned and crossed the street to a different pay phone and called Bob, his sponsor.

"Listen, Bob, I'll be out of town for a while. I don't want you to think that I'm screwing up or anything," Larry told him. "I'm not even sure I'll be able to call you."

"Sounds like you're working again."

"Bob, you know I can't say anything about it. I'll try to stay sober and remember what you have taught me," Larry sounded pained. This was a harder call than he thought it would be.

"Okay, Larry, just remember that AA is everywhere, and that you can make your own choices. I'll put you in my prayers and see you when you come back." Bob sounded full of emotion. He felt that Larry wasn't strong enough to make it through an undercover assignment with out drinking and it showed. Larry thought about calling Jackie, but he wasn't sure if it was the right thing to do and he was out of quarters.

Back in room 112, Larry sat back against the wall and reviewed his busy day. No real amends to make today. The meeting with Captain Moffit, the long drive, then the encounter in the restaurant with the tall cowboy, and, now the loneliness of knowing it was unlikely he'd see another friendly face for several weeks. This brought his thoughts back to Jackie. Had she really said that she was attracted to him? Last night's date with her was enough to spark all kinds of inviting daydreams. She really was about the most fascinating woman he had ever encountered. He said a little prayer. "God, show me your will and protect me if I'm worthy. Help me come out of this alive, 'cause I think you have given me and Jackie some unfinished business. Give me the power to do your will. Amen." He reached to the night-stand for his Big Book, but it wasn't there. Larry turned out the light and stared at the dark.

In the morning, Larry called the contact number at nine o'clock. The phone was answered by a youthful woman, identifying the phone as a Treasury Department field office. Larry hung up the phone immediately. Angry that an undercover operation would be put together so amateurishly. He walked a couple of blocks while reviewing the situation in his head, then stopped and called again from a different phone. This time he left a blind message for the red headed treasury man to call the pay phone number.

"It's your dime," Larry said when the phone rang.

"This is special agent Jerry Smith. I assume this is Larry, can I have your location and room phone number?"

"It would be really dumb to admit that on an open line and no you can't have that information. So far you are not impressing me, pal. You had better come up with something a little more professional or this conversation is over," Larry scorned.

"What do you want me to say?" Pleaded the red head. "I'm sorry. I'm not as experienced in this type of an operation as you are. We need your services. Are you going to help us?"

Larry held the phone against his chest for a moment to think. He had a bad feeling about this one. "What the hell. I'm already here," he said, "Here's what we need to do. One, don't call me from the office again. Two, don't ask me to call there again. Three go find a cell phone that is not related to you or your job and barrow it for a while. Four, start thinking about my survival, not your convenience. Five, meet me at a place called "Wally's", over by Fort Bliss at six o'clock on Friday evening."

"But that's three days from now," the agent wined. "How will I know you?"

"You sent me the ID stuff, remember. And Smith, don't make me wait," Larry hung up the phone.

Larry didn't see any reason to change motels yet. He walked back and got the van to run errands. First, he visited Ralph's Guns and purchased a enough ammunition to refill the guns he had been given. Then rented time on Ralph's shooting range to test the weapons. Next he went to the library to use a computer. With his special police codes, he was able to find Tom Sullivan's records and data files. After scanning this, he printed out key pages. Next he ran the plates on the van to find out who's car he was driving. It was registered to

Shirley Sullivan, the wife. Larry thought the van seemed out of character for a "made man". He dug a little deeper and found that Sully drove a pickup similar to the one Chuck Norris used in his TV show. The truck had been repossessed when Tom had gone to jail. Sullivan's jacket also revealed that his wife had recently died of cancer. The record photo of Sully showed that he and Larry were similar in looks. Sullivan was Italian and Irish. He didn't have a beard but Larry thought that worked for him instead of against him. He could explain the beard by being away for awhile and it would help cover any facial differences.

After the library, Larry found a truck dealer and rented a silver-gray four by four pickup for two months. In the processes he discovered that Sully's credit cards had lots of room to charge anything he needed. Next he rented a garage at a Store-N-Lock and put the van in it. To complete the cover, he then stopped at a western store and purchased two leather vests, one black and one brown, a new Angelo styled black Stetson hat and a belt with Sully custom stamped on the back.

Back at room 112, Larry studied all the new information and then burned it as before. Still no knowledge of whether or not Sully was an AA criminal or not. He decided to pass on the restaurant at the motel and go down the street to a fast food joint. As he was parking the pick up, an old red Chevy Silverado pulled up. Climbing out of the new arrival was the smiling face of Trevor.

"Well, howdy there, Sully," Trevor's grin was infectious. "That looks like a pretty fine ride you got there."

"I just got it today," replied Larry, "These new ones are comfortable, but those old Chevy's never die."

"You got that right. I've had this old girl since she was a youngster. Bought her new in nineteen hundred and seventy-seven. Let's go inside and I'll buy you a burger. We can swap truck stories." Trevor had trapped Larry with a "good old boy" custom and American tradition.

Once again, Larry was happy to see a sobriety friend, but still worried about his cover. He really needed a meeting, however, this good-natured cowboy would have to do. Anytime two sober drunks get together, the conversation always turns to an AA related topics.

As they sat down with their soft drinks and cheese burgers, Larry heard himself blurt out. "I forgot to pack my Big Book for this business trip. You wouldn't have a spare you could lone me, would you, T?"

"Why certainly, I pick them up in garage sales and second hand stores all the time. You never know when you might need one for some poor suffering alcoholic." Trevor was up and headed for his Chevy before Larry could respond.

Returning to his cheeseburger, Trevor handed Larry a used Big Book without the dust cover. "Keep it. I've got three more under the seat of the Chevy. Hell of deal, the way this AA thing works, ain't it? One minute you're trying to be alone and sad, the next you're having burgers with an alkie like me." Trevor had a way of zinging to the core. Larry had heard a lot of sponsors were that way. Bob certainly was. He responded.

"You were right the other night, Trevor. It is hard to be a stranger. My higher power is revealing more to me all the time about how this works. Did I look sad to you when you drove up?"

"No. Not really. I just have a feeling that you ain't been on too many business trips since your sobriety date. That's how this disease works. It looks for a weak spot and tries to make you feel sorry for yourself. The more you start saying "poor me", the closer you are to saying "pour me a drink". And no matter what you may tell yourself, no one really likes to be alone."

Larry was really starting to like this guy. "What do you think a person should do if he can't get to meetings."

Trevor finished his burger and took a long drink of cola. "Well, it starts with your spiritual condition. Do what it takes to keep that channel open to your higher power. The serenity prayer helps me a lot to get through tough situations. Sticking my nose in the Big Book helps, too. To get that daily reprieve from this disease, you need to get up in the morning and make a choice not to take a drink, no matter what. Even if your butt falls off."

Trevor and Larry went on talking for about an hour on how to do the program when you are out of your own town. Trevor was interesting to talk to, inserting enough of his own personal stories to keep the subject away from Larry's life. As he drove back to room 112, Larry realized that he had the same good feeling that he gets by going to a regular meeting. He spent the evening reading in the book. Looking for a way to handle this assignment and his sobriety without ending up dead, either way.

Friday, Larry moved his base to El Paso, checking in to a deluxe suite at the Holiday Inn. It was a much better room than number 112 at the City Center Motel. Three rooms with a wet bar and a basket of fruit. There are fancier hotels in the area, but the Holiday Inn had easy access, and he could park the truck in view of his window. Sully was used to the best in his line of work, so, Larry thought the suite added a nice touch to the cover.

Al Bennette was suppose to be in Mexico, doing business in and through Juarez and El Paso. This operation was going to take Larry across the border, so it was time to go see Fast Eddie. Eddie was a tall three hundred pound Mexican who owned the best hamburger place in west Texas. On the side, he also owned a bail bond company that his brother and two cousins operated. As skip tracers, they worked across the border most of the time. The 'Feds' often used them to bring out bad guys. Usually, they would kidnap the subject and kick him out of a van on the bridge just over the half way mark. The FBI or Marshals or whoever, would make a clean arrest on the American side. A rich big name criminal like Bennette was going to take a lot more finesse.

Eddie was behind the grill, preparing for the lunch rush. He was one of two people in El Paso who new Larry was a cop.

"Hey, amigo," Eddie bellowed as he rushed around the counter to shake Larry's hand. "Como esta, hombre. How are you?" He leaned in close as he shook hands. "Do you have a new name this trip?"

"Call me Sully," Larry said softly, then louder, "Muy bien, my friend. How's the burger business?"

"Let us have some coffee and catch up. Do you have time, Sully?" Eddie walked Larry to a corner booth and signaled the waitress who was already bringing two cups and a thermo pot full of coffee. She knew her boss often talked business from the booth and didn't allow interruptions. For Eddie, everything was serious business. His success rate for skip tracing was among the best, and he knew absolutely everything that happened on this part of the border.

"What's up this trip, uh….Sully? It is good to see you, but you're wearing a very serious look. By the way, the beard's a nice touch."

Larry grinned at his old friend. "Does this look better? I guess I'm kind of a new man, Eddie. That last deal with Bumper Blue just about did me in. Lost my wife, my self-respect and almost my job. I'm better now. Haven't had a drink in almost ten months."

"No disrespect to Sally, but she wasn't really cut out to be a cops wife. Even after, what was it, seven years, she just didn't have the hard side to her that it takes to live with what you do." Eddie had been to Larry's wedding and several camping trips with Larry and Sally. "If a cop's mate is too soft, the fear and worry will just eat them alive. Seen it happen to lots of nice couples."

"Well, maybe there is something there, but I have to take responsibility for my part. It was mostly the drinking that brought out all these defects of character that I have. After I sobered up, we tried some therapy. It was just too late for us. I did too much damage." Other than Bob, Eddie was the only person in the world that Larry could really open up to.

"Now you are sounding like one of those AA folks. Is that what you've been doing with your time?" Eddie pulled a six year coin from his pocket and laid it on the table.

"Eddie, why didn't you tell me you were AA? I could've used the help."

"Oh, you wouldn't have listened, even to an old friend like me. You were so full of pride and fear the past few years. All you seemed to be doing was trying to control all the people, places and things. You not only took the job home with you, you loaded it in the damn bus and tried to drive it through the front door, metaphorically speaking. And if you have done some AA, you know that an alcoholic should never drive the bus. Especially when they're drunk." Eddie would never let it be known that he was the one who called Captain Moffit, and the AA people in Albuquerque to get Larry started in the program.

"You don't know how good it makes me feel to know you understand," Larry was wearing a genuine smile now. "I need some help in Mexico, Eddie."

"Sure, amigo, that's why you're here. Who are you looking for this time?" Eddie leaned his huge frame across the table.

"His name is Bennette, Al Bennette. He's running a counterfeit store for the Italians from Chicago." The tone of the conversation was suddenly serious as Larry proceeded. "This guy's hard to catch up with. They want me to get shipping information and the whereabouts of both Bennette and the plates. I've got to start somewhere, so here I am. I figure, if you don't know about it, it's probably not real."

"Yeah, I've heard of this gringo. He has a hacienda down at Chihuahua. The locals call him "El Cigarro," We thought it might be phony money. He wasn't hiring enough local people to be processing drugs."

Larry was impressed. "That was easy. Has he been that obvious, to attract attention to what he's doing?"

"No," answered Eddie, "my uncle is his gardener."

Larry chuckled. It always amazed him, how well connected Fast Eddie was. Ed had a huge family that watched both sides of the border for him. "I think I'm going to need an introduction to Al Bennette or one of his top men. Before I go there, I need to get as much information about the set up as I can. I'll know more after I meet with my contact tonight. Can you get me a guide for Juarez? Somebody who knows more than they should, and can be trusted."

"No problemo, amigo. Call me tomorrow morning and I will arrange for my nephew to show you the back side of Juarez. His name is Francisco, everyone calls him Cisco. He works with us when we cross the border. He's a good kid, tries to stay up on everything from the border to Chihuahua."

More family. Not a surprise. "That sounds good to me. I'll probably want meet a bad guy in Juarez or El Paso and let him take me to Chihuahua, but it will be great if Cisco can help me get connected."

"Okay, jefe, call me about this time tomorrow and I'll have something for you." Eddie extended his giant hand for another shake. Don't forget, one day at a time."

"Thanks mi amigo, it's been great seeing you again," Larry said loud enough for others to perceive them as the old friends that they were.

"Vía Con Dios, Sully," Eddie announced to the room. Walking back to the kitchen, he noticed the first customer of the day, a tall cowboy with a leathered face, ordering a cheeseburger.

Larry noticed Trevor also, but the cowboy didn't seem to see him, so Larry left out the side entrance, not wanting to mix business and sobriety any more than he had to. The odds of Trevor being here exactly at this time were almost incomputable. Larry let a mild warning scribble across his consciousness.

Later that evening, Larry stepped through the doorway of "Wally's Cowboy Bar and Grill". He was dressed in his new hat, leather vest and custom belt, all on top of his regular solid color button down shirt, wrangler jeans and boots. Allowing his eyes to adjust to the din, he slowly removed his chrome-plated aviator sunglasses that he had purchased to enhance his tough guy image. About fifty men, mostly dressed in work clothes and cowboy boots were present, along with a table of soldiers from the base that were wearing their fatigues. Here and there he saw a Stetson or straw hat, but mostly sweat stained ball caps . Larry knew this was a working mans bar and not the sort of place where city slickers would be likely to be found. Still, every bar had it's code. Larry knew the rules in this one. Even with an old pair of jeans and deliberately scuffed boots, he was almost too clean for "Wally's". He asked for a coke at the bar and carried it over to a table, facing away from the door. The point is to blend in. Those desperadoes in the movies who sit with there back to the wall, stick out like a soar thumb. He pulled the lime green "REAL COWBOYS DON'T LINE DANCE" button out of his vest pocket and laid it on the table. It was meant to be worn as his identifier. No way was he going to wear such a stupid thing in a place as ruff as "Wally's". After a few minutes the red head showed up in a bad J C Penny's suit and carrying a brown brief case. Larry watched covertly as he drew stares at the bar while ordering a yuppie water. The bar tender just laughed and said, "We haven't had that here since the last remodel job." After looking around to notice the scared 1940's interior, the red head chuckled at the joke and settled for a Heineken.

Turning from the bar, Jerry Smith spotted the lime green button on the table and his face lit up instantly, like a Roman candle. He tried to catch Larry's eye. "This just ain't gunna work," Larry mumbled to himself. The red head was crossing the bar brief case in one hand and Heineken in the other. Larry tried to ignore him.

Gliding up to the table, the red head spoke as he started to sit. "Hi! I'm Jerry. You look like you could use some company."

Larry exploded from the table, grabbing Jerry's tie and pulling his youthful face eye to eye. "Leave me alone you red headed peacock," he yelled. Then under his breath he said, "Men's room, now." Then throwing him backward, he again raised his voice. "I don't care what you're selling, pretty boy. I don't need it." All who noticed, basically everyone, laughed as Jerry scrambled to his feet, drenched with his own beer, and went through the door marked, "BUCKS", before the beer bottle had quit spinning on the floor.

Larry waited at the table shaking his head and mumbling to himself like a lot of drunk cowboys do. When it appeared that all had put the incident behind them, he shuffled to the men's room. Inside Jerry was still combing his hair. "What the hell are you trying to do, get me killed? Who put you in an undercover situation, anyway? Don't you think you should at least try to be a little discrete?"

"Hey, lighten up. I thought I would come as an IRS agent," Jerry quipped.

"What's that a joke? My life is on the line here and you want to get us both killed, then joke about it? The key word there is agent! I've never seen anybody who looks more like a federal agent than you do. You put me in this situation, so you're going to have to suffer the consequences. Meet me at "Denny's" restaurant, off Interstate-10 at eight in the morning." With that Larry popped Jerry cleanly in the side of his nose. As the blood gushed from his face, Larry kneed him in the groin, grabbed his shoulder and threw him through the door. As he came out of the restroom, Larry's size ten boot knocked him to the floor with a blow to the backside. Stepping over the red head, Larry scowled at the bar and barked, "you better start watching the type of people you let in here, Wally," then stomped through the exit.

At the end of the bar, Trevor looked up from his coffee cup and grinned.

"Good morning, my name is Tina and I'm your waitress this morning. Would you like some coffee?" Larry nodded as he sat down in the booth with Jerry Smith.

Jerry ordered coffee and sweet rolls for both of them. The cavalier spark was gone from his eyes and he had medical adhesive tape across his nose. His brief case was open on the seat.

"I'm not going to apologize for last night. You may not understand, but the way you handled yourself in that bar scared the crap out of me. I've seen operatives killed for grinning at the wrong time." Larry's tone was subdued and serious, but not angry. You forced me into making a show to protect my cover."

"Don't worry about it. It works good with Tom Sullivan's character. You are right. This is my first undercover action. I didn't know we had to be so careful here in El Paso when the perps are in Mexico," Jerry explained.

"Where are you from?" queried Larry.

"Originally, Ohio, but my office is in Seattle," said Jerry. "To answer your next question, the Seattle office was flooded with this phony money a few weeks ago. They have had me tracking the source for most of the last month. So, here we are."

"How did you find me?" Larry knew how the system worked. He needed just to be sure.

"I knew this was going to Mexico and I asked for a Spanish speaking covert operative. The Tom Sullivan thing was somebody else's idea. We found him in jail, ready to cooperate. Although he is a made man in the mob, he never felt loyalty to the Chicago mob, his parent family. They needed someone to take a fall on the Vegas tax case, and chose him. Tom's wife was in the final stages of cancer and he wasn't too happy about missing their last few months together. True love, you know."

The kids story had a good start for his cover identity, however, experience told Larry to beware when wearing someone else's skin. "So Sully is mad at his bosses. Do we know if that will last? What's in it for Sullivan? What happens to him when this is over?"

Jerry pulled a manila envelope from his brief case and removed a stack of papers and photographs. "They sent me this documentation so you would know the truth about his case. Here are his wife's death certificate, his early release forms from prison, his application-stamped accepted-for the witness protection program under the RICO act, and his affidavit claiming the facts of his mob life to be true."

Larry examined the documents, checking for the proper seals and stamps. Larry was no amateur. They papers looked good, so he nodded agreement.

"Okay. Here's the complete Tom Sullivan bio-sheet. Pictures of his house, wife, dog, cars, vacations, and a few mob associates. As far as we know, none of the latter are in this area." Jerry winced at the vagueness of the last statement. Larry shot him a look that would break glass.

Immediately, Larry was taken by two things in the pictures. First how happy Tom and Shirley looked as a couple, and second, how much he and Sully really did look alike. He handed the photos and papers back to the agent, keeping the biographical sheet to memorize and burn later.

"Thanks, Mr. Smith. So how do you want me to play this." Larry sounded friendlier now.

"They said you were a tough one to convince. Here is the way we see it. You can improvise anything you want. As you say, your butt's on he line. Tom's job was to over- see the Phoenix gambling and to act as a go between for the mob and the Indian gambling operations. We have him out on an early parole due to overcrowding. Instead of reporting back to his bosses in Las Vegas, he, that is you, get wind of the counterfeiting and show up here. The reason for being here, is that he is trying to broker a money laundering deal between the Mafia and the Indians. We think it's a good cover story. If successful, it would be a big boost to his crime career, and show his bosses that all is forgiven," Jerry ran out of air.

"Sounds plausible. Who came up with that idea?" Larry asked.

"It was Tom Sullivan's idea. He said shady money deals were already in place with the American Natives back in Oklahoma and a few other places," answered Jerry.

"Did he say exactly how it works?" Larry was thinking there was hope for this mission after all.

Smith replied. "It's really simple. The Indian casinos buy the phony money at thirty-five to fifty cents on the dollar. Then they give it out in winnings. It's good business for the casinos because they can give more generous winnings, which brings in more business. People love to win cash. The Indian reservations are considered sovereign states, so it is a little harder for Treasury and the IRS to keep tabs on everything. We do, but if they don't want to cooperate there isn't too much we can do. I mean, have you ever tried to push an Indian to get what you want?"

"Yeah," Larry said. "My mother."

"Oops. I'm sorry," Jerry cringed.

"That's okay," stated Larry. "Your perception is right. Native Americans can be so stubborn, you would think they had tree roots instead of legs. My mother was Choctaw, and my father was an Irish police sergeant in Oklahoma city. She used to take me to the reservation to visit relatives, but I grew up a city boy. So, my job is to pretend to bargain the amount the Indians will purchase and for how much on the dollar. Do you have information on the casinos for me?"

Jerry took a few more papers out of the brief case. "Here are the names of the casinos, the lists of tribal committee members in charge, and so on. And this page has all the financial information like how much cash they should be willing to buy and how much they can probably afford to pay."

"Are these figure fictitious, or did Tom supply them?" Larry asked.

"They came from Mr. Sullivan. Our boys compared them to what the FBI and IRS know. They Looked good as far as we could tell." Jerry was glad this mornings briefing was going better than his previous experiences with the undercover operative. "By the way, here is my card with the cell phone number you asked me for, on the back. The cell belongs to an office girl's mother. We bought her a new one with all the fancy gimmicks on it as a trade."

"Okay, Mr. Smith, you're done here. You can leave now," Larry said abruptly.

The agents face fell. "When will we meet again?"

"No offense, Jerry, but if I do my job, never."

"But I thought we would be working together on this," Jerry protested.

"We are," Larry said, "you're part is to stand by the phone and supply me with information when I need it. And if everything goes to hell, I may need extraction, you know, rescue. You can't do either of these if you are tagging along. Besides, I really believe you might get killed. So, just get up and walk out now and I'll call you. I'll even spring for the coffee and rolls."

The agent packed his brief case and stood up. Looked as if he were going to say something then walked out the door. Larry was relieved to see him go. He didn't seem like too bad a guy, but all that inexperience was hard on the nerves. These were dangerous people and a lot of money was involved. There was no doubt in Larry's mind that they would kill at the drop of a hat in this operation, especially in Mexico, where officials can be bought for the price of a used Chevy Suburban. He studied the information and drank another cup of coffee. There was a lot to consider. The source of this information seemed reliable, unless Tom Sullivan had a bigger plan to take out a bunch of 'Feds'. Not likely. That was a point to worry about, however, Larry knew that an operation like this would have experts and shrinks going over every detail, but it was a mystery why they sent this young inexperienced agent to handle such big case. Al Bennette was not a small fish to land. The only explanation Larry could conclude, was that more agents were in the area, maybe even under cover, and the kid was just a front man for the Treasury Department and the FBI. "On yeah, that makes sense," he said out loud to himself. Federal agents were always over-doing it. Layered investigations and undercover people bumping into each other unaware of the consequences. Just then a familiar face slid into the booth. It was Trevor again. Larry looked up with a blank expression, his hand discretely turning the papers over to hide the contents.

"Hiya, Sully," Trevor said with that twinkle in his eye. "Fancy meeting you again, and in another restaurant. Can I buy you breakfast or have you eaten already? How's sobriety today?"

"My sobriety is fine, and no thanks on the food. I just had a sweet roll," answered Larry, trying to be friendly, but feeling a bit invaded. He hated to mix business with non-business. This cowboy had just showed up at the wrong time. Such things could be dangerous, and now he was wondering about Trevor's accidental meetings. He decided to take a leap with his undercover story. He had to find a way for Trevor to fit the operation. This was Trevor's terrain, Larry didn't think this guy was following him because he was careful to check for such things. It would be hard to believe Trevor was a bad guy, if he was he probably wouldn't be so obvious. Probably a nosy cop of some sort.

"I just finished a business meeting that didn't go well and I'm in sort of a bad mood."

"Well, such things happen in life. Anything you want to talk about?" Trevor sounded too convincing to be anything other than what he seemed to be, even if Larry had a hard time believing in coincidence.

"I just had a meeting with my parole officer. I didn't tell you before that I found AA in prison." Larry started the "cover-lie" as he called them. Not hard to do and make believable; you just had to remember the details you told to whom. "He wants me to hurry up and get a job, but my wife passed away while I was in jail and I have a good chunk of insurance money to live on." The best way to tell a cover-lie was to wrap the truth and the lie together in the same blanket.

"So you're not a businessman from Phoenix on a trip?" Trevor still had that sly grin on his face.

"Sorry about the lie, Trevor, but after being inside, it's hard to know what to say to someone. I'm from Phoenix, all-right, they just released me into this area to keep me away from my old friends."

"Were you in for drugs?" Trevor queried. "That seems to be common among AA people these days."

Trevor was making this easy. Larry joined the evolving lie.

"Yeah, just some small time dealing, they kicked me out early for overcrowding. But You know, after getting in AA, all that criminal stuff is gone. At the time I was busted, I didn't think I was doing much wrong. Of course, I was drunk most the time anyhow."

"Sure, I can relate, they night I jumped the cop, it was just for laughs. Never thought I'd be going up the river," Trevor chuckled. He had a way of putting Larry's mind at ease. "I don't wanna be pushy, but here's a list of local meetings. Sounds to me like you could use a few." Trevor pushed a pamphlet sized paper over to Larry.

"Thanks, man," Larry picked it up and put it with the other pages that he had folded and paper clipped when Trevor arrived. He looked at his watch and exclaimed, "Gotta go, Trevor, my PO set up a damn job interview for me this morning. Sorry, I'll see you around, maybe at a meeting." Larry stood and put the money for the ticket on the table.

"That's okay," Trevor said with sincerity, "my phone number is on the back of that meeting list. Call anytime, Sully."

Larry walked out, climbed into the four-by-four and drove away. Trevor drank another cup of coffee and grinned.

Larry drove back to the Holiday Inn and called Fast Eddie from a phone in the lobby. "Hey, Eddie this Sully, anything for me, yet?"

"Si, amigo, my nephew will meet you on the bridge around noon tomorrow. He can guide you like all the other gringo touristas. He said his bike is bright green with a white basket. He knows what you are driving, so he'll find you."

"Okay, Eddie. Thanks for your help. Do I owe any money?", said Larry.

"Na, Cisco's already on my payroll. Just don't forget favors for favors, Señor," Eddie laughed.

"Bueno, my friend. It's deal," Larry hung up with a smile.

The best news he had in this case, was his friend Fast Eddie being in the program. He went to his room to relax and study the new information. Then he read a little in the Big Book that he got from Trevor. That reminded him of the lie he told to Trevor. It was about time to clear that up, so he called Smiths' cell phone number. It was answered on the first ring. Larry said he had an important question for his cover story, "Did Tom Sullivan attend AA meetings in prison?" The red head promised to find out and hung up, only to call back two minutes later with confirmation. This news relieved Larry's mind for a few moments, then he realized that he hadn't told Jerry Smith where he was staying or what his number was. That proved it. The 'Feds' had a surveillance team on him. He didn't like that, but it was common in these kinds of cases. He just hoped they didn't follow him across the border.

Later that night with his meditation done and prayers said, he lay in the dark and thought about Jackie back in Albuquerque; wondering if she was doing okay. He missed her and wished they'd had more time together before this operation had started. His life with his ex-wife seemed like a far off dream now. Somewhere in his memory was the feeling of comfort and companionship that marriage had once offered him. It had been too long since he had felt the soft touch of a woman who cared. Even in his marriage, the last few years felt cold and lonely. Being gone so much, he and Sally were like strangers when he was home and as her anger turned to disgust, and her love turned to disillusionment and he turned more inward. And turned more to the bottle. His failed relationship was not an excuse for his drinking, it was just a natural by-product.

It can be a lonely thing to sober up and realize that everyone is gone. Imagining how it would be with Jackie was a compulsion that he wasn't sure he should allow. Was she right for him? Was he good enough for her? Could he be a good man for her? Would someone as well put together emotionally as she seemed to be, lower herself far enough to tolerate someone like him? Larry had no answers. Sleep was difficult. He hugged a pillow and waited for the sandman to come, but he must have forgot Larry. He got up about one o'clock and got dressed. Thought he'd get a cup of coffee or something. The coffee shop in the motel was closed, only the bar was opened. He peaked inside and decided to go for a walk instead. At an all night mini-mart, he bought a pack of gum and got a stack of quarters. He found a pay phone and dialed Jackie's number. The answering machine picked up on the fifth ring. It was good to hear her voice even if she wasn't really there.

"Hi there 'Double L', it's me. Ah, I ah, let's see.....I'm out of town....ah....I'm working. Remember our discussion at dinner? Anyway, I enjoyed our date and I'll see ya when I get back." The machine cut him off. He felt more lonely than ever now. Why wasn't she home? Probably just doing overtime in the ER. She said that she works a lot.

CHAPTER 4: JACKIE

She sat in as many AA meetings as she could, hoping to see Larry again. Her schedule at University Hospital had been killer lately. Way too many people showing up in the ER with over-doses, violent wounds and car wrecks. Jackie never thought about the irony of the situation, her a recovering alcoholic taking care of all these people with alcohol and drug related problems. She just took it as the least she could do to repay for the damage she had caused when she still drank and used too many prescription drugs. Jackie hadn't told anyone except her sponsor about the drugs. Most of them she had stolen from the hospital that she used to work in, down in Las Cruses. She had been quietly fired when she was discovered by a doctor, how ever it didn't show up on her record. She guessed that she wasn't the only one dipping in the medicine cabinet. So, someone had covered her theft so that they could go on doing the same thing.

Meetings came and went. Several days had gone by and still no Larry. All she had to hang on to was a goodnight kiss and a message on her answering machine. So here she was, in her regular noon meeting, almost two weeks later, trying to focus on one day at a time and the best cliché of all, "keep it simple stupid"! It wasn't simple to forget about Larry. Some how he had touched her soul and she just didn't understand why. Her sponsor had said that sometimes understanding was the booby prize.

Jackie's attention came back into focus with Rita S., a mousy thirty year old with a quiet voice and messy pale brown hair, she was talking about her experience, strength and hope.

"And I also felt shame for my family. My beautiful little girl, my mom, my husband and all those who cared about me," Rita's face was a picture of self-contempt.

"When I lost my man and my child all in the same week, I realized that maybe, I did have a bad problem. Even then, it still took over a year to find help. My life just went spiraling down until there wasn't anything left. No job, no family, no place to live, no car, no money, no self-respect and no faith. Then a wonderful lady saw me steal a beer from a table in the truck stop and approached me. She asked me two questions. One, why didn't I steal the food when I so obviously needed it? And two, did I think my actions were normal for an intelligent adult woman?"

"I wanted to cry but no tears would come. Right then and there, I knew I was spiritually busted. My response to her was almost animal like. I don't remember what I said, but she listened and then put her arm around me, put me in her car and drove me to a detoxification center. Three days later I got on my knees and asked God to forgive me and to help me find my way back to humanity." Rita

35

continued with tears in her voice, "That lady saved my life and the only thing she ever has said about it is "but for the grace of God, go I.""

"This program works. I know it does because they let me see my daughter, Shelly, yesterday. After a year and ten months of a sober life, that was a miracle to me. Every day in this twelve step program I do three things that work for me. I pray for knowledge of God's will, I admit that I'm an alcoholic, and I try to help someone without their knowing it. This program works when you work it. Thanks for letting me share. Sorry for the tears."

Immediately relating to Rita's story, Jackie remembered her own feelings of despair and emptiness at the time of her introduction to AA. She had wandered north to Albuquerque after being fired in Las Cruces. Things went from bad to worse. It took too much time to find a new job. Later she realized that she attended several job interviews with booze on her breath. Most people have a hard time trusting an openly drunk nurse. She had to sell her nice car to afford to live in a motel room. Then her purse was stolen when she was drunk at a bar in Old Town. Like most drunks, she didn't trust anyone else, including banks, so all the money she possessed was in her purse. Thirty days later, she was allowing men take her home from bars just so she could have a shower and maybe breakfast, before they got tired of her slobbery, drunken ways. Home was a sixty-nine Plymouth station wagon. Her wardrobe dwindled down to one dress, blue jeans, and a couple of T-shirts. Out of money and the proverbial rope, she was forced into temporary sobriety for a few days. Halfway coming to her senses, she cleaned up in a gas station and tried one more time for a job, this time at University Hospital.

Katherine was working in the personnel office at that time. She interviewed Jackie the same as all the other applicants, then she got up and shut the door. "Listen, sister," she said, "I work with all kinds of people and I've got to tell you, the nurse on this application is not the person I see before me. Let me tell you something. I was a bad drunk for many years and now I'm free of that obsession. I'm living proof that you don't have to remain a slave to that way of life. If you are ready to admit you have a problem, there is a way you can be helped. If not, I wish you luck and goodbye."

The tears came as a flood. Jackie just sat and cried for what seem like an eternity. That night, she went to her first AA meeting and slept on Katherine's sofa. It was a couple of months until Katherine determined that Jackie was strong enough to hold down a job.

At the Sunshine Café, Jackie sat, remembering a guy in the hospital the night before. Stories like his were all too common. Mangle body on a gurney-product of two much alcohol and a fast car. Being a trauma nurse was not an easy job sometimes. His broken a body arrived in such bad condition he looked more like road kill than a forty year old man. Along with smell of bodily fluids was that unmistakable odor of alcohol. Near death experiences happen every day because of booze and drugs. The question she asked herself often these days was, would she see Larry in a similar circumstance. After this much time, some of the program people who knew him were saying that he must have gone back out drinking. After all, he was a regular, often doing two or three meetings a day. A slip they call it. Jackie thought the word slip was a silly way to describe an event that often caused human beings to loose their lives. She wanted to have faith that he was keeping his sobriety in tact. Jackie was hesitant to talk about Larry because he was so secretive about his work. The last thing she would want would be to responsible for getting him in trouble or hurt. There was no way to tell if what she might say could effect his life, so it was better not to join in any of the gossip. Of course, Katherine was different, she could be trusted and Jackie was starting to fill up with emotions. Jackie's lack of information on the subject was turning into worry. Too much worry became depression and a black cloud started forming in her mind.

By the time Katherine showed up, Jackie had worked herself into a foul blue-gray mood. Katherine, after so many years of sponsoring and caring about other women in the program, had no problem diagnosing a problem of the heart. She quietly seated herself and casually asked, "Do you wish to talk about it or are you going to keep that heavy blue funk all to yourself?"

"Hi Katherine," Jackie took a ragged breath, "You know, after a while all the drunks and drugies get to me. I know I'm one too, but why do so many people feel they must throw their lives away? You would think a few light bulbs would go on."

"Hey, Jackie," Katherine answered, "You are a nurse. An RN. You have dealt with these facts for years. What's really bugging you? There must something more. Is this about that Larry guy again?"

"Kathy, you work in the office. Most of the people you see are excited about having a baby or are waving insurance forms in your face," snapped Jackie, "you don't see the daily trauma cases missing body parts, and hardly recognizable has humans. I've seen just too many of them and they remind me how short and precious our lives are."

Rather large for a Navajo woman, Katherine was about two hundred pounds and five foot nine. Her long shiny blue-black hair, even in a traditional braid, hung to her ample waste. Enormous silver trimmed glasses graced her high cheekbones, giving her soft dark eyes an appearance of intense wisdom. One of her more endearing habits was her need to wear as much Indian jewelry as she could. She was blessed with Native American natural beauty and armed with both a psychology degree and eleven years of sobriety.

Kathy backed off a little physically and softened her tone. "My aren't we testy today. I don't need to remind you that you asked to work in the trauma unit, against my advice, I might add. Sweetie, if the fire is too hot, don't stand so close to the flame. Ask for a transfer. You have a position at the hospital, they won't want to risk loosing you. At least take some time off for Gods sake. You don't want to hear it, but this is about that guy at some level. Ever sense he disappeared you have been working eighty to a hundred hours a week. Working yourself to death isn't the way to get over some man. They're all pretty much the same you know. All ego, attitude and sex drive."

"Larry's not like that!" Jackie offered almost too quickly.

"You see. I was right again, kiddo," Katherine said. "It is about him, isn't it. Jackie, the guy's a drunk. And he went and did what drunks do. Just forget him and get on with your life. You don't even know the guy, really!"

"Careful my friend, you might hurt my feelings, and in my condition that could be fatal." Jackie responded with a chuckle, and a large smile for her sponsor. "He may be just a 'guy' to you, but he seems to be a bit more to me, now doesn't he? I may not know where he lives or what his occupation is, but I know good when I see it and that little inner child voice of mine says that I want him. All kinds of things could have happened to him besides getting drunk. Aren't you pre-judging him a little? I've heard the gossip and I don't think it's right."

Katherine had her just where she wanted her. "So you were sitting here all blue because you are afraid that I'm right and he will show up on a gurney in the Trauma center. Projecting your fears onto this relationship, you insist on having, will only breed resentments. And resentments do what to us? They get us drunk. You know better than to let yourself get too lonely, tired and hungry. I know you aren't getting enough rest, with all the hours you work. I bet you haven't had a good meal all week. Let's order steaks. My treat."

"Okay, okay, you win as always Katherine, how did you get to be so smart?"

"Lots of mistakes, is there anyway else to learn?" Katherine smiled an motioned for a waiter. "Promise me you will take a little time off and find something else to think about. I know this new girl who needs a sponsor. The two of you would be compatible, and you would have an excuse to dwell on something other than work, or a guy you may never see again. What do you say, Jackie? I have her number right here. We could go over to her house and I could introduce you right after our meal.

"You never give up, do you Kathy?" Jackie resigned.

No, not on you I don't," said Katherine warmly, "lets order."

Jackie resigned herself to doing what was suggested by her sponsor. She decided that she just needed to turn this Larry business over to God, and let go of the outcome.

The next step for Jackie was to cut her schedule at University Hospital. It wasn't an easy thing to do. Once the supervisors start to depend on someone like her, they don't want to let up. She did manage to cut her schedule back to the seventy to eighty hour range. She could have cut it a bit more, but she was getting some flight time in as a substitute flight nurse on the helicopter, and she just loved to fly.

Another positive step was to take on the sponsee that Katherine had suggested. The girl was Suzie G. from the noon meetings. Jackie found that they were both nurses at University Hospital. Suzie was an LPN that worked in the maternity ward on the same shift as Jackie. The two of them arranged to take breaks at about the same time, when they could, which allowed time nearly every day for sobriety discussions. Jackie felt that her record as a sponsor was tarnished after two of her sponsees had slipped and not come back to the program. However, her own sponsor reminded her that it is a program of progress, not perfection.

On a lunch break, Jackie and Suzie sat in the commissary pushing unidentifiable casserole around on paper plates. Suzie was about twelve years younger than Jackie and although she seemed competent as a nurse, she was apparently just as interested in the extra-curricular activities around the hospital. University Hospital is just what the name says, a university with lots of young men and women destined to be successful in the field of medicine. A virtual 'candy store' for a young beauty like Suzie on the prowl. With her blond hair, expensive make-up and tight uniforms, she never failed to get the second glance. If Jackie could get her to think about sobriety as much as she thought about men, there might be hope for her, but, sobriety was a struggle for Suzie. Jackie felt that the young nurse had just not reached her bottom, yet. It was simply just not important enough for her to stay sober. Jackie pledged to try and get though to her anyway. If nothing else, maybe she could stop her from falling too hard on her pretty face, or maybe, make it easier for her to get back up once she did trip and stumble.

"I just don't get all the contradictions in this stuff," wined Suzie, with a mock pout on her face, "like, how come everyone says I have to change all my friends and the places I go for fun, when in the Big Book, it says just the opposite? And don't just say one of those damn clichés like "more will be revealed."

Jackie took a deep breath to reinforce her patience. Suzie wined too much. Jackie felt like telling her to just stop wining and grow up. All those clichés were important pieces of wisdom. Instead she said, "Well, you have to learn to sort through the Big Book and what you hear at meetings, and find the things that will keep you sober. My suggestion is that you not run from your friends until you know whether or not they are willing to help. Your drinking friends do not have to quit drinking for you to be friends, however, they do have to respect what you are going through and who you are becoming. Just the act of getting sober will change most of your relationships. Some for the good and some for the worse. I certainly wouldn't go out to a drinking party or a bar with your old friends until you have enough time and understanding to "meet any condition" as they say. And then only if there was a good reason to be there."

"I want to know when this spiritual stuff is gonna happen. I'm young and I don't want to sit around being bored all the time. I need to get back to having some kind of fun. You say I shouldn't even date." As she spoke, Suzie's lack of maturity was so obvious that Jackie couldn't help 'rolling' her eyes.

"No, I said to be careful with your personal relationships for a while. Many a love life gone wrong has pushed a newly sober person back into the bottle."

"I don't want to drink, Jackie, but I don't want to be a sad old maid, either." Suzie's wine was about all Jackie could stand today and it was hard not to take that last line personally. But then again, Suzie had no way of knowing about Jackie's love-life. In fact, Jackie probably wouldn't be thinking about how lonely she was if Larry hadn't come along.

"So you think that I'm a sad old maid?"

Suzie squirmed in her plastic chair. "Well, not really, I mean…. You're not like me. You're so, so, adult."

"Mmm, maybe you could use a little of that in your life?" Jackie tied to make it into a joke, but overall this conversation wasn't going too well. Her own mind was distracted. She could sit here and spout AA stuff all day, however, if her mind was not on it, it wasn't really fair to Suzie. It's hard to give advice when you feel off center in your own life.

"Look," Jackie said, "you can choose your friends and you can choose your circumstances, but be aware that friends and circumstances come with consequences attached. So, be careful. Be sure. And most of all, be true to yourself. The sober self, that's sitting here right now, not the old self that drank and used. Are you getting the message Suzie, or do you need a little more air for your head?"

"I think I've just been insulted. I'll let you know after this refill." Suzie picked up a notepad and started waving it frantically at her ear.

"Do you get what I'm saying, sweets?" Asked Jackie with a more pleasant tone.

Suzie put down the notepad. "Yes, I hear ya, mother Jackie. I'm not all blonde hair and big chest you know, and I don't use white-out on my computer screen, either!"

"Sometimes I just don't know if you understand that this is a life or death program. I don't mean to be sarcastic with you. I just want you to think about the choices you must make everyday."

"You're right, Jackie, AA saved my life, I have no doubt about that. Like everyone says, "do what is suggested, and the promises will come true." And I want to live in a life where I'm not full of fear and loathing." Suzie settled back with that glazed over look that seems only to happen to the young and innocent.

Jackie was satisfied for the moment that Suzie would try to be good for another day or so. "Let's meet for breakfast and go to the noon meeting tomorrow," she said. "If you can drag your young butt out of bed early enough."

"Okay," Suzie answered, "but if I turn into an old maid before I turn thirty, you are in trouble."

Alone in the night, Jackie sat on her bed. The longer she was sober, it seemed the more she did not understand the life she and her God had created. Long ago, she learned not to pray for God to fix her life, only for knowledge of God's will for her, and the power to carry it out. Jackie did feel better after taking Katherine's advice, however, in these quiet moments alone, the feelings of longing for Larry had no boundary or explanation. Was Larry the "right man" for her? Where was he now? Was he doing something dangerous? She could imagine his soft romantic touch. The taste of his lips, and the strength of his arms seem real. She missed his presence, and didn't understand why she felt so close to him so fast. Jackie whispered a quiet prayer.

"God grant me the serenity to accept this lonely life, the courage to go on and face my character defects daily, and the wisdom to know your will for me today and tomorrow. Please show me your will about Larry. It has been several weeks and he still haunts my mind. Is this love or loneliness. If my character defects are blocking this part of my life, please show me the path to remove those certain defects. Amen."

No immediate answer came. Jackie, sat still for a few moments until the tears burned her face. Wiping away those tears with the sleeve of her robe, she adjusted the light by her bed, picked up her Big Book and leaned back to read herself to sleep.

CHAPTER 5: THE GERMAN

Standing on a balcony of Pancho Villas' mansion, now called, 'The Museum of the Revolution', the German surveyed the city of Chihuahua. A romantic lover of art, culture and historical architecture, he had grown so very fond of this city of a half million hard working and proud people. Ciudad Chihuahua's history ran deep in the culture of Mexico. At the confluence of the Sacramento and Chaviscar rivers, it had been a natural historical meeting place for many of the areas two hundred tribes of Native Americans. A place where even the fierce Apache warriors had been subdued by the more passive tribes with their easy going attitudes. Later, when the Spanish came, it became a wealthy mining city with a richer than rich upper society, supported by a population of hearty, honest workers.

Most of the magnificent buildings had been built by the proud Indian craftsmen, to the specifications of the Spanish Governors and priests. These marvels have been maintained and honored by the local rescendants, so most of them remained in wonderful condition; undamaged by the weather, wars and pollution that had ravaged much of Europe's architecture. The beautiful Cathedral of pink stone was the masterpiece of the town and reigned like royalty over the other great buildings; Federal Palace, Plaza Hidalgo and Maseo Casa de Juarez, where the historical Mexican hero had resided during the revolution, while Maximilian held Mexico City for a while.

The German sighed. For two years he had been here in the "Lady of the Desert", as they called her. He would always think of Chihuahua as a woman, beautiful, full of charm and grace. And sexy. His Petra had been all those things before she had died, without warning, in that auto crash, taking his love and her family inheritance with her. He had not known another woman since. Seven long years of tortuous memories, abated only by this beautiful city.

Soon after Petra's death, he had switched from a serious artist to a counterfeiter. At first it was signatures and official documents. Easy, quick money. Then replicas of fine art. Rewarding but slow money. Soon enough, he drifted into currency and printing. Actually, fine art on very small formats with a huge profit. There are dozens of countries where the technology isn't in place to catch bad money on the streets. Using only the nick-name of "Wolf", which was derived from his real middle name, Lieth Wolfgang Von Stein, he worked is way through the currency of lesser nations. Always perfecting his skills. Making a profit, then selling off the plates and inking formulas and moving up the scale until he was in international money. Having done deutschemarks, rubles, pesos, lira, and yen, he bought a Hacienda here in Ciudad Chihuahua and started on the big one-the currency of the United States Of America.

"Señor," Carlos, the Germans' body guard and driver, interrupted his thoughts. "It is time to go, Señor." Von Stein nodded to the large Mexican-Indian. From his size and features, he guessed he was a mixture of Apache, Raramuri, and Spanish, washed together on the stones of time. Powerful and serious, Carlos had worked as a mercenary in Africa and Columbia before returning to his roots. In this country, a body guard was needed, not because the German was a small man, most of the locals were small in stature, but, because Von Stein insisted on a lifestyle of the rich. He was an easy target to pick out in a crowd with his pale bald head, full gray mustache, and glasses. He was accustomed to wearing fine clothes and smoked a pipe which served to further his arrogant, aristocratic European attitude. He attended social functions in his armored Mercedes, that Carlos had obtained for him from the estate of a late drug dealer, making him an even bigger target for Mexican banditos. But no worries with Carlos around.

As he was driven from the center of the city, his mind shifted to the upcoming meeting. Lieth didn't like doing business with the Mafia, and this man Bennette, repulsed his sensibilities. The man was an aging knuckle-dragger, vulgar in all the ways of the civilized. Loud and obnoxious, he drank too much, cursed like a devil and made awful crude comments about the women servants in his house. Then there was that damned fat cigar that he used almost as a weapon, waving it in the faces of the meek, gesturing with it to make a point and blowing fowl smelling smoke in an opponents eyes. Carlos had told him that Bennette liked to burn people with it when he wanted information, or when a prostitute was less than pleasing.

The Italian had invaded the city a year ago, and immediately started looking for illegal operations to profit from. He had procured a large hacienda, through forceful tactics, and guarded it with a small force of third rate thugs and bandits. After a time he had discovered that the "Wolf", the infamous counterfeiter, was a fellow resident of Chihuahua.

The first time the Italian wanted to meet the "Wolf", he sent a couple of thugs in a jeep to request Von Steins' presence by strong arm tactics. Carlos interrupted the quasi kidnapping and had a grand old time with the interlopers. It wasn't much of a challenge for a man with Carlos' training, but after inflicting several broken bones, he tied the unconscious victims into the front seats of their Jeep Wrangler and had his cousins' wrecker service tow it back to Bennette's hacienda. Realizing that he had underestimated Von Stein, Al Bennette sent a formal invitation for dinner the next time. Although Bennette's table manners were something that the German would like to forget, the meeting had some merit. An arrangement was made for a trial distribution of Von Stein's fifty dollar bills.

It had been nearly two months time since the distribution of the phony fifties. The German assumed that it was time for a progress report and some negotiations. Getting into bed with the Mafia was serious business, not to be taken lightly. Lieth Von Stein had spent many hours going over his needs, desires, motivations and plans for the future. He had over a million US dollars of real money tucked away in a numbered account. In Mexico, he could maintain his lifestyle for a long time on a million dollars. So, it wasn't just the money. Pride of his art was foremost in his mind. Producing counterfeit bills had become his new art form. His new passion. If he quit counterfeiting, could he return to his previous art form of oil painting? Had he ever been a really great painter? He wondered. He knew without a doubt that he was a great counterfeiter. A master of an art form that few had tried. The Mafia could handle the distribution of his new art into North America and beyond. But what did they want besides money? The Mob always wanted, no, demanded, more than just money from those who dared to do business with them.

Driving up the small hill that Bennette's hacienda crowned, both Carlos and the German took inventory of the rag-tag squad of guards. They seemed to be of different ethnic backgrounds. A red head with freckles and bad teeth manned the front gate, still wearing a cast on his wrist. When he spoke to them, his accent was Irish. Two Hispanics were stationed on the roof of the house, dressed in jungle fatigues. Another three odd looking characters covered the front of the house. It was assumed that more were in the back. Carlos noted that all of the guards carried AKMS rifles, the newer folding stock version of the AK47, that all the bad guys used in American movies. He could also see an assortment of hand guns in both shoulder and belt holsters. None of this worried Carlos. Usually with these types of people, the more guns they had, the less training they had. An AKMS in an untrained hand was an inaccurate weapon. And few people spent the practice time and volume of rounds that it takes to be proficient with a pistol. Carlos was an exception to this rule. He had convinced the German of the value of experience and Von Stein was glad to provide a shooting range in the barn, where Carlos fired about 1000 rounds a week. Being always prepared for anything, Carlos was also a black belt in two different disciplines of martial arts. His weapon of choice was the Beretta M9, nine millimeter, currently in use by the US Army. The M9 was a reliable gun from the factory, however, Carlos owned five of them that had been reworked by a master gunsmith. He wore a custom made shoulder holster that held one M9 upside down, in the back, below his shoulder-blades and one under his left arm. On his belt, in the back, he had a total of eight clips for the Berettas. Each clip held eight rounds and although a lot of shooters these days go for the larger clip guns like the Beretta 92FS model that holds fifteen rounds, he felt the extra weight would where you down in a protracted gun battle. With the two loaded guns and extra clips he could shoot eighty times. Attached inside his dark gray jacket were two small flash-bang grenades. It was an uncomfortable array to wear, but comfort wasn't his concern.

The other three M9 handguns were concealed inside the car. One in each font door panel and one stuffed in-between the back seats.

As they approached the house, Carlos took one of the concealed guns from the car and tucked it in the front of his belt. After letting the German out of the back seat, he pulled the gun, worked the slide and moved the safety to the ready position. Holding the gun with both hands, but down in a non-threatening manner, they approached the door. At least three AK rifles were trained on them. Bennette's number one, an Italian called Bruno, came through the door to greet them.

"I'll take that," Bruno gruffed. As he reached for the gun, Carlos simply sidestepped leaving Bruno in an off-balanced lurch.

As the Mafioso recovered his balance, Lieth Von Stein spoke. "Now be fair, Bruno, you have several loaded weapons trained on us. Don't agitate my man and start a blood bath. We came for business and dinner, not to shoot people. Carlos, safety the weapon please."

The body guard made a show of moving the selector to the safe position but continued to hold the M9 with his hands folded in front of him. As they followed the Italian into the large house, a ruckus was underway in a room to the side. A middle aged woman in a black and white maids' uniform was tied to a kitchen chair. Her dress was ripped open in the front exposing her chest. From a distance of seventeen feet, Carlos and the German could see two round welts on her breast from fresh burns. Al Bennette was leaning in close to her, cigar in the corner of his mouth. Among a dozen or so swear words, he was yelling about missing cufflinks. Reaching into his back pocket, he pulled a small plastic garbage bag. As he circled behind her he blew cigar smoke into the bag several times and then pulled the bag tight over the woman's head. The woman stiffened with terror. In a moment, Bennette removed the bag and left the woman gasping and sobbing. "Tell the bitch to pass the word to her friends. We don't want no stealin' at Hacienda Bennette," the mobster laughed. "Put her back to work, but in the kitchen this time. If she don't like it, kill her whole damn family." A thug cut the ropes with a switch blade and dragged the hysterical woman off into the house.

Bennette turned and greeted his guests. "Well, my business partner has arrived. Come on in Mr. Wolf. Let's have a drink. Sorry about the show, good help is hard to get these days. This used to be her family's house, so the bitch thinks she can do what she wants."

Carlos made a growling noise. Von Stein said, "You run your house and I'll run mine. It is none of my affair." He then handed Bennette the bottle of ninety year old scotch he had carried in. "This is for you, Al, but we are not partners, yet."

"Sure we are, we just ain't set no terms yet." Bennette was wearing a white Mexican wedding shirt with a salsa stain on his large stomach. He took the bottle, opened and poured himself a shot. After downing the shot, he poured himself a double scotch on the rocks and a scotch and soda for his guest. Carlos was ignored by the Italian, just as he was used to ignoring his own men.

"I'm as hungry as a maggot in a dumpster. Come an' eat, then we can talk 'bout our money."

At the dinner table, two beautiful young Mexican girls of about fifteen years were seated; one on each side of the table dressed in revealing evening gowns. They looked straight ahead. Never smiled or spoke and only pushed green salad around on their plates. Obviously, fear and drugs ruled their lives. After dinner's small talk, Al offered one of the girls to the German. As he declined, Carlos, standing in a corner, winced. Both girls were his cousins, and he ached for the chance to free them from this white devil. But, he was working now. His personal interests would have to wait.

The view from Al Bennette's verandah was breathtaking in the late evening. Ciudad Chihuahua twinkled to life under the great expanse of the stars. The German had a coldness that allowed him to distance himself from the conduct of this vile man. Business was business, and Von Stein had to do business with a lot of low life types since he had started his new career. Even though this Italian exhibited just about the worst example of human behavior, Von Stein knew he could tolerate him long enough to get paid.

Bennette let go a long loud belch. "Well now, Mr. Wolf, this looks like the time of day for us t'do some business. How ya doin' with them other bills?"

"Some are ready and some are not," answered Von Stein, "how did the distribution go?"

"My people were pleased," Bennette continued. "Most of it went to the pacific northwest. They didn't want to put it in their own back yard until they were sure that your stuff was good. The word is that we're gunna do business with ya, but the top guys in the organization want some guarantees."

The German was already braced for this part of the negotiation. "I assume they're not talking about a written contract. What is it that they require. I'm a reasonable man."

"It's all 'bout control, ya know," Bennette said. "They ain't gunna be happy if you're sellin' your bills t'anyone else but me."

"So they would like an exclusive for North America. I will not have a problem with that." Von Stein expected that, and the United States of America is the hardest place in the world to pass American currency. "I can give you my word on that right now, assuming we come to terms on the price."

"Ya, okay, but there's more." Bennette poured himself another drink and held the bottle out for Von Stein who declined. "We don't want you sellin' no phony money in Europe either."

Von Stein really did not care about Europe. In some European countries, the technology for discovering bad money was even more advanced than the USA.

The German knew everything about passing counterfeit bills. With the introduction of the new US bills that contained tracking data strips, Von Stein thought it would be a good time to retire from this business. However, he needed to broker a profitable deal to retire on. No-one would expect him to sell this set of counterfeit plates, the most valuable in all the world, but that is what he intended to do. He had finished the full set three months earlier and had been stock-piling money every since. After selling the plates to the Mafia, he was going to sell the millions that he had stockpiled to drug cartels in Columbia and El Salvador. American money, even phony money, was the currency of the drug traffickers. The old style money, and his set of plates, should have eight to ten years of use before the new money replaced all American currency.

"Yes, I can live with that. Any other terms they wish to impose?" said the German.

"One more," Bennette wore an evil grin. "They would like me to keep the plates in my safe here at Hacienda Bennette."

Von Stein waited for a while before answering, to give the impression of discomfort. "What if that is not acceptable?"

"Listen Wolf, don'tcha understand who I represent? These are dangerous men. They don't like to hear the word no." Bennette was slurring his words, his temper and his voice were rising.

"Oh let me assure you, Mr. Bennette, there is no reason to raise your voice and make threats." The German chuckled inside at how easy it is to manipulate this barbarian.

"As I said before, I am a reasonable man. My decision depends on how much money can they use and how much are they willing to pay?"

Bennette felt he was winning and calmed himself. "Twelve cents on the dollar for tens and twenties, and nine cents on the dollar for fifties and hundreds. The good news is that they can use all ya can make in the next couple'a years."

At those rates, Von Stein would have to produce about twenty million dollars in counterfeit to make the two more million he felt he needed to retire. "Can you guarantee a usage figure, say thirty million in counterfeit over two years?"

"That's no problemo, but we keep the plates on the days you're not printing and one of my men has to be there when you are, to insure our agreement, you understand."

The German smiled. "That will be acceptable to me Mr. Bennette, with just one modification. I will only allow you to keep the back side of the plates in your safe. To insure our agreement, you understand?"

It was Bennette's turn to smile, a victorious smile. He would rather have done something to hurt this arrogant European, but he had to answer to his bosses as well, and all their demands had been met. After they had reaped the rewards of his Chihuahua deal, the bosses would have no objection to the German's disposal. "We can call that a deal, Mr. Wolf. When can you deliver some goods?"

"I can have the first million next week, half in large bills and half in small. Can you have a ninety thousand dollar payment by then?" The German wanted to test the agreement right away.

"Sure, sure. Like I said no problemo, my friend, but I thought you said all the plates weren't finished?" Bennette didn't like being lied to.

"Just a few finishing touches on the ten dollar plates. I can have the bills ready one week from today," Von Stein lied and promised. He leaned forward and lowered his voice to a respectful tone. "Al, I would like you to take a proposition to your people."

Bennette raised his voice again. "Now don't ya try t'wiggle outta da deal!"

"No, no. A deal is a deal and I know we are both men of our word," the German pleaded. "I would like to propose that your people buy the whole operation. I have five Mexicans trained to do the printing, drying and bundling. The operation is set up in a secret location. All the machines, the building, trained workers and the full set of plates for three million American deposited in my Caiman Island account."

Somewhere in Bennette's mind, a cash register bell had just dinged. Bennette could afford that much money from his personal accounts. He could buy the set up, sell to the bosses and they would never be the wiser. "Okay, Wolf, I'll take it to the bosses. It sounds reasonable to me, but I'm just the middle man, ya know. I'll see if we can get their answer by next week. I gotta tell ya, them guys like t'dicker on the price of things they buy."

"I will look forward to a counter offer," Von Stein felt relieved. This wasn't as hard as he had thought it would be. "I'll have that drink with you now, and we can toast to being partners."

"Bueno," Bennette said, and then poured two more glasses, spilling some of the expensive scotch as he did so.

Under the stars of Chihuahua, they sat and drank. The German smoked his pipe and listened while the Italian rambled drunkenly on about the good old days in the Chicago mob. After about an hour, Bennette passed out and Bruno showed Von Stein and his body guard out. Nothing was said about the hosts' drunken behavior. Bruno had seen it all before.

In the sleek Mercedes, crossing the city, Von Stein discussed the evening with his body guard. "Did you know those girls at dinner, Carlos?"

"They are both cousins of mine, Señor Wolf. How did you know? It's not professional of me to acknowledge my personal life when I am working," Carlos was genuinely embarrassed.

"It is all right Carlos. We are friends, too, are we not? I have noticed that when you are agitated, you stand in a more defensive posture. Your left foot is slightly forward, your hip is swiveled inward, and the gun that you usually point down, is level, ready for action. And I could swear that a few times, you have actually growled like an animal." The German smiled as a friend, but Carlos was still in a bothered state.

"I'll try to do better, Señor Wolf.", was his answer.

Von Stein felt compassion for this man. Bennette was a beast, and to have family members at the whim of such a devil would be hard. Especially when you had the talents that Carlos possessed. "I know it will be hard for you, mi amigo, but no matter how much we dislike this despicable man, we can't do anything against him before we get paid. You heard everything Carlos, do you think we will get paid?"

The bodyguard hesitated for a moment, then spoke respectfully. "Señor Wolf, business is business, and it is your business, not mine. I will do what ever you say, the honorable person that you are, earns my loyalty."

Von Stein ran his thin hand over his smooth bald head. "Gracias amigo, thank you for the complement. Pull over up there by the cathedral, I wish to speak to you face to face."

Carlos complied. The beautiful baroque eighteenth century church, with it's German pipe organ and it's Italian sculptures, was fitting place for a serious conversation. The German opened his own door and stepped out. Leaning against the car, facing the church, he lit his pipe. The bodyguard came to his side and lit a cigarette.

"Do you like this city, Carlos?" Von Stein gestured around them with his meerschaum white briar pipe.

"It is the home I knew as a boy señor Wolf." Carlos seldom said anything personal. "The passion for ones' home grows with time, and my people are very passionate about this place."

"Yes, your people built this beautiful city. They should be proud. I know they have tried to take care of this city in spite of the outside influences that have threatened this way of life. Even with the latest surge of American industrialization, most of your people have adapted without giving up their old values." As the German spoke, Carlos felt pride for this place and his Mexican/Indian heritage. "This Italian and his Mafia are a cancer in our city. Already they have been changing the crime scene from one of desperate peasants to hardened criminals. The people of the state of Chihuahua can deal with a few bandits and minor crimes, but these Italians bring death and misery to Pancho Villa's very doorstep."

"Si, I too am aware of the growing problems in Chihuahua," Carlos said as he instinctively looked behind them. "There is talk on the streets that El Cigarro is buying off the city and state officials. If he spends enough money, he will be unstoppable."

"Carlos, I could never ask you to murder anyone, but what we are doing now is very dangerous. These people will want to kill me as soon as I am not useful to them. I would like to make you a full partner in my business. That means that when we get paid, you will be worth over a million US dollars. All I ask is that you keep us alive until the money is in the bank. After that, if you feel you have to take certain steps to insure our safety and cleanse Chihuahua of this cancer, well, that is up to you." Von Stein wiped a spot off his glasses with his shirt and turned to look Carlos eye to eye with out his glasses. The Mexican could see the honor and respect in the Germans eyes.

"Bueno, Señor Wolf. Mucho gracias. I understand and I'll be ready. But I would do these things anyway, it's my job." Carlos took a deep breath and slowly extended his hand.

With a firm shake, Von Stein confirmed his commitment. "You are a good man Carlos. You deserve this. I do not want either of us to spend our lives looking over our shoulders. And Chihuahua is my home too."

They took their respective places in the Mercedes and drove on into the summer night. Each man lost in his own version of the future, their fates sealed together by respect and common purpose.

CHAPTER 6: MEXICO

In spite of his Mexican/American, sort of ethnic appearance, and his working knowledge of the Spanish language, Larry was still just another 'gringo' crossing the Rio Grande River into Mexico. A real Mexican has an attitude that is almost genetic. This is not a reference to the Hollywood stereo type, although you are certain to find the 'East LA' types in major cities. Most Mexican people are proud, hard working and honest. Politics and economics have ravaged their culture and their country. Many Mexican families from the countries interior, send a family member or two across to 'Del Norte' or the north, to earn money to send back for food and necessities. On even a minimum wage job in America, a young man can send enough money home to sustain five people. Latino refuges from the neighboring countries to the south, have flooded Mexico with cheap labor and a transient population. The boarder cities like Tijuana, Juarez, Acuna, and Matamoros have swollen way past any type of control by the Mexican government. A man who was once a lawyer in El Salvador may live in a cardboard shack next to former politician from Columbia, who, with his family, live in a broken down car body that has a ragged tarp over it. Across from them can be a fourteen year old mother who sold her body to survive last year, and sells it this year to feed her baby. All border towns have this type of neighborhood. Most of those people want to get across the border to work and feed their families, not to hang out on street corners, sell drugs and steal cars, as Hollywood would have Americans believe. Minor crimes in border towns go unpunished unless they occur in front of a law officer. Most of the transient population will do almost anything to feed themselves. It is into this environment that Larry must go to get information.

Larry turned onto Santa Fe street in El Paso and proceeded south to the river. As he crossed over to Mexico, he put on his game face. Like turning up a volume knob, all of his senses became more aware. Many years of undercover experience had taught him to see all, know all and predict all. During a simple act like driving down a street, Larry was considering who was in the vehicles around him, where the best escape route was on every block, what could possibly go wrong, and if it did go wrong, what action could he take to survive. If you could go in with guns and karate chops like they do in the movies, it would be a lot easier. But in real undercover work, especially the type of deep cover that Larry specialized in, you had to think. Think, think, think. Make plans and adapt to the out come. An operative who does not understand this type of work, never makes it home. In this case, he had learned where the bad guy is located, but he couldn't just go charging in like Chuck Norris. He would have to meet some of the right people, and a few wrong ones. Then he would have to establish credibility; prove his word. If he survived all of that, then he could work his way through a bunch of lessor criminals until he was introduced to the man in question, Al Bennette. To do all of this takes time, lots of time, but the first step was to meet Francisco.

As he came off the bridge onto Avenue Juarez, Larry saw the young men on bicycles. There were seven of them out this morning. What they do is to ride up to your window and offer themselves as a guide. If you accept, then you follow them in your automobile to your desired location. Of coarse, they will take you to a shop or restaurant where they have an agreement in place. If you spend money, then they get a percentage. Sometimes they will even help you shop and will make a big show of bargaining with the shop keeper, forcing him to slash the prices until you are willing to part with your American cash. Usually, if you knew how to bargain and spoke Spanish, you could get it at about one third of what the guide had settled for, but the system served a good purpose. The gringo touristas enjoyed the show and usually thought they had the best deal and a few Mexican families get fed on the gringo dollar.

A bicycle slid up to his window from behind the truck while he was at the first stop light. Larry had his window down.

"Good morning Señor," the cyclist said in with a heavy accent. "My name is Cisco. I want to be your guide today Señor. For one American dollar I will take you to see anything you want in Jaurez. Just one dollar and you can follow my fine green bike anywhere you like."

Larry handed him a dollar and instructed Cisco to find a parking place downtown. The young Mexican took off down Avenue Juarez at break-neck speed. His bike weaving in and out of the many cars on the street. Every few hundred feet, he would turn to see that he hadn't lost the silver pickup in the heavy traffic. When Larry finally caught up with him, Cisco had his bike on the curb, motioning frantically to Larry to park. Jumping out of the four-by-four, Larry thanked the cyclist and told him he would like to hire him for the whole day in a voice loud enough to be heard by others on the street. After agreeing to a price of six dollars for the day, Cisco settled his bicycle into the back of the pickup and climbed into the cab.

"Thank you for helping me maintain my cover," Cisco said in perfect English. "My uncle was right, you are a professional. Good to meet you Mr. Sullivan. What can I really help you with?"

Larry answered. "Just call me Sully every chance you get, to begin with. Nice to meet you too, Francisco. Fast Eddie and I go way back. He said you had your ear to the ground over here and could be trusted. Instruct me around the city for a while so we can talk in the truck."

Cisco gave him some instructions and Larry started driving. He had driven in Ciudad Juarez many times but a moving truck was a good place to talk business and keep Cisco's' cover.

"I need to know everything I can about an Italian named Al Bennette and his dirty money operation in Ciudad Chihuahua. We have plenty of time. No need to rush this. It is not life or death, unless we get caught." Larry swerved hard to miss a crazy driver who turned left in front of him across two lanes of traffic. Driving in any large Mexican city is an exciting experience. "The object is to eventually get a meeting with this Italian guy."

"I get it, Sully. You want to go through all the hoops to get to the top so you have a cover story with local history. Very smart Señor," Cisco grinned.

"That's right Cisco. What I need the most from you is help in finding the right bad hombres that will lead up the correct trail. Maybe we should try to buy some phony money, just to sow a few seeds. What do you think?" said Larry.

Cisco knew, as Larry did, that phony money was a commodity on the Mexican border, just like sugar or marijuana. "Well, I have a cousin that has a boyfriend, his name is Ricardo, he might know someone. The man in Juarez who fences the large amounts of bad cash to the drug dealers and such is called El Gordo, the fat man. We can't go to him at this level, you are right Sully. It takes time and the right contacts to reach someone like El Gordo."

"When can we start working up the food chain?" Larry asked.

Cisco instructed Larry to pull over by an open air market. "Give me twenty dollars, Sully."

Larry did as directed and Cisco jumped out of the truck and disappeared into the maze of booths. Soon he reappeared with a bag of food and a pretty Mexican woman about thirty years old pushing a soft drink cart. Cisco laid the sack on the hood of the truck and tore it open, revealing four huge tamales. Larry got out and joined him.

"Señor Sully, this is my cousin, Maria, She has been overpaid for the drinks so you may ask her for information about Ricardo." Cisco reached into the cart and pulled out a Jarritos Mandarina soft drink. Larry did the same.

"Hola, Maria, habla ingles?" Larry smiled at the woman.

"Yes, Señor Sully, I am an American. I just work here. I own ten of these carts around the city." Maria was obviously proud of her business.

"That's very good, Maria. You must hear a lot of things in this business," stated Larry. "Does Ricardo run with a bad crowd?"

"Sometimes he does things for Groupa Diablo. They are a gang in the city. They sell women, drugs and extort money from business people like myself." Maria didn't sound agitated with this.

"Por favor, Señorita. What is your connection to this Ricardo?" asked Larry. Maria smiled devilishly. "We are special friends, and Groupa Diablo leave me and my carts alone."

Larry understood that she paid for protection with her body. She seemed like a nice woman, he hoped it was worth it to her. "How could I meet this man?"

Maria said, "I'll see what I can do for you. Come see me tomorrow. My cart will be on the north side of Plaza de Americas."

"Muchas gracias, Maria. Hasta mañana," Larry said in poorly accented Spanish.

"De nada," She said over her shoulder as she and the cart disappeared into the market.

Larry turned to Cisco who was deep into his second tamale. "What's next?"

"You gunna eat that?" asked Cisco, gesturing at the remaining tamale. Larry shook his head and smiled. "If you're gunna do business in Mexico, you better get a hotel room here, Sully. It's a thing of respect for our country. These people don't ever really trust a gringo, you know."

"Okay, how about Hotel Plaza Juarez?" Larry finished his tamale and downed the soft drink. "Can you find someone to watch the truck so it doesn't get stolen?"

"Sure Señor Sully, I have a cousin who'll do that all week for just fifty dollars." Cisco and Larry both laughed. Larry felt instantly comfortable with this skinny, fast talking kid. Cisco seemed to know his stuff and with Fast Eddie's recommendation, he gave the kid more trust than he would usually afford a stranger, but then again, Larry was becoming more trusting than he used to be. In the back of his mind, it bothered him a little. He hoped he hadn't lost his instinctual 'edge' for this type of work.

The next day Larry checked out of the Holiday Inn at five in the morning, hoping to shake his government tale. He drove across the Bridge of the Americas which emptied into downtown Juarez at the Plaza de las Americas. The hotel was on the side of the plaza, on the corner of Avenues Lincoln and Cayoacan. Larry parked the big silver pickup in the hotel lot. When he got out of the cab, a man popped up out of nowhere. As Larry instinctively reached for a gun, the man quickly explained, in broken English, that Cisco had hired him to watch the truck. Larry just shook his head and went into the lobby to register. At the door to the suite, as he was about to pay the bellhop, Cisco showed up, grabbed his wallet and paid the man.

"You must be careful, Señor Sully, not to tip too much. It will give the locals the wrong impression of you. Buenos dias, amigo. You come early." Said Cisco.

"Yes," replied Larry. "But you were apparently here first."

"I slept in the servants quarters, they called me when you arrived. I have friends and cousins in all the hotels. My real business is information. It helps to have lots of friends, and the rest I pay," claimed Cisco.

"So, which side of the boarder do you live on?" asked Larry.

Cisco plopped down in a swivel chair and put his tennis shoes on the oak and glass coffee table. He seemed to change from grinning Mexican street youth to confident businessman in a blink of an eye. "I know I can trust you, Sully, or what ever your name is. I know it's not Tom Sullivan because I checked him out on the internet. He just got out of prison. And I know I can trust you because I remember seeing your picture on my uncles' wall. Younger, no beard and wearing a cops dress uniform at a wedding."

"Well, Cisco, that's an impressive bit of police work. Are you sure you're not a cop yourself?" Larry's voice was smooth and friendly but his eyes had turned to steel.

"No, I'm part of Fast Eddies bail bond company. I'm a skip tracer on this side of the boarder. To answer your first question, I live on the streets down here most of the time, but I do own a nice house in Las Cruces, New Mexico. I legally have dual citizenship, thanks to our co-operative governments. Uncle Edwardo wants me to go all the way with you on this. Be your back up, not only your guide. I can handle myself in a fight and I'm up to speed on a lot of common weapons."

Larry pulled the Glock from under his leather vest and laid it on the table. One of the nice things about Mexico is that you can bring almost anything into Mexico, it's crossing into the US that is a hassle. He then sat on the sofa and put his feet on the glass across from Cisco's. A gun on a table would intimidate most people. This was a new twist. Larry always worked alone. Probably the only person in the whole world that Larry trusted enough to change his MO, was Fast Eddie. This kid seemed all-right. It's hard to trust someone with your life, but he did need his services to operate inside Mexico. Larry's Spanish was good but not good enough to pass as a Mexican down here. He didn't expect any violence, however, when the Mafia is involved, anything can happen and it would be nice not to die alone in the desert. Larry stared at Cisco for a couple more minutes just to see what the kid was made of. Cisco never flinched. Finally, Larry grinned and said, "Let's go down stairs and rustle up some Huevos Rancheros."

In the hotel coffee shop Larry ordered huevos rancheros and Cisco ordered something that looked more like dinner than breakfast and smelled like menudo.

Larry opened the conversation in a friendly tone. "Listen, Cisco, you work under cover, like I do, so you know how hard it is to have a partner. There is a whole cover scheme in place here. I will fill you in but not in the open like this. We'll talk in the truck later. Just maintain the guide routine, show me the sights and we will work on the case as we go. Just no serious talk in the open. It's too easy to listen these days with all the electronics. Okay?"

"Muy bien, Señor Sully." The grinning street guide was back with a heavy accent. Cisco leaned forward. "Do you know that hombre over there with the two senoritas? He was at the market place yesterday. Maybe he is a gringo friend, eh?"

Larry turned to see Trevor paying for his meal with a pretty girl on each arm. Mixed emotions flooded his conciseness. The first thought was that Trevor was definitely following him. The second thought was that an AA buddy was near, and that was comforting. If he was following, he was probably a federal officer, if not it was just God's way of reminding him to stay sober. He tried not to make eye contact, but Trevor turned and came to the table.

"Howdy Sully, doin' a little sight seeing?" Trevor's' good mood was almost infectious. "Hey, I know it's probably been a while, you want one of these, on me?" He pulled the two girls closer to the table.

"No thanks, T, I got the whole day planned. This is my guide, Cisco," Larry motioned to his new partner.

"Mucho gusto, Señor Cisco." Trevor tipped his cowboy hat. "Well, my friends, I got business to attend to. Maybe I'll catch up with you later Sully. Hasta luego." Trevor spun on his heal and headed upstairs with the two señoritas giggling as they went.

"I think I've seen that man many times in Juarez. Drives an old pickup." Said Cisco. "If he's a cop, he's local and well established in his cover. If he is a bad guy, I can put the word out for information on him. We will know in a couple of days."

"Don't worry about Trevor," Larry said. "He is just someone I met a few days ago in a restaurant. He's nothing." Larry wanted to believe his words, but Trevor was starting to show up just one too many times. If he was a fed, there was no need to blow his cover. If Trevor was on the wrong teem, it would work for Larry to establish his credibility. "Show me some sights, Cisco." Larry put on his Stetson and they headed for the truck.

Cisco and Larry drove around the city for a while discussing the operation. Larry explained the Tom Sullivan cover and how he perceived the progression of the operation. He had reoccurring thoughts about why he was trusting this guy. He had never trusted anyone in the field with so much information before. His conclusion was that he had changed, probably because of AA, and now he trusted some people a little more. He just hoped it didn't get him killed.

Before the border was created, El Paso-Juarez was one city called El Paso Del Norte or The Passage to the North and later as two cities, El Paso, Texas and Del Norte, Mexico. In the 1860's it was renamed in honor of Benito Juarez, the Native American (Zapotee tribe) who became president of Mexico after a series of revolutions. Benito Juarez was called the emancipator of the spirit-the Mexican Abraham Lincoln. The city has a certain amount of old world charm and sites to see, the Guadalupe Mission built in 1659, Plaza of the Founder, Plaza de Armas, the open air markets with arts and crafts on Sixteenth of September Avenue and the Museum of History located in the old customs building. As a city of fifty thousand, it would be quite comfortable and charming, however, somehow, another three-quarters of a million people were jammed into the city. People are everywhere. They sleep everywhere, eat everywhere, defecate everywhere. And most of them just waiting to cross the border. There are people in Juarez from every part of Mexico and Central America. Larry, being half Indian himself, felt a bond with the poor masses. He didn't see them as Mexicans, only as people. His people; Native American Indian people. He wished he had time to learn more of their culture and history. The history of a people conquered many times, who have been oppressed for most of the past four hundred years. The Spaniards, the Church, the French, and a series of corrupted governments have held these people down. And now, it is the very change that they need so badly that oppresses them . Maybe catching a major crook or two would help in some small way.

Late in the morning they parked back at the hotel and walked into the Plaza de Americas looking for Maria and her vending cart. They found her instructing a new employee, a country girl of about fourteen who was in awe of the big city and very grateful to have a job.

"Hola Maria. Como esta usted?" Larry thought it would be polite to try to speak Spanish when he could.

"Buenos dias. Muy bien, gracias, Señor Sully," Maria replied. "You be careful with that bad Spanish, greetings are okay, but don't try to say anything meaningful. You could be misunderstood. Maybe even shot for it," She laughed.

"Do you have any news for us?" Cisco asked. He was eyeing the pretty employee.

Maria took a few steps away from the cart. "Isn't she a little young, even for you, cousin? Ricardo says he will meet you for a price, but not in the city. He will see you this afternoon at Paquime."

"No problem," Said Cisco. "Did you tell him how to recognize us?" He walked back to the cart and purchased a soda from the girl, looking her in the eye and making her blush.

"Everyone knows the silver pickup by now, Cisco. You know how fast news travels in the underground." Maria had her hands on her hips and her head thrown back. "Now get out of her before this innocent girl gets any ideas."

"Muchos gracias." Larry liked this woman with the strong character.

"De nada, Señor Sully," she took his hand. "You can trust my cousin with your business, but you have watch him around the pretty senoritas."

Cisco said his good-byes and they walked back to the hotel. So far, so good thought Larry. It just takes time.

There was a knock on the door. Larry looked at the clock. It was four o'clock already. He had dozed off reading in the Big Book that Trevor had given him.. He was studying pages 100 and 101 about being ready to meet any situation. He thought that being prepared to meet any situation was very real at this time. So far, he hadn't been tempted to drink, but this assignment was just beginning. The book says it's all about maintaining a spiritual condition. Well, no time for prayers now. He and Cisco had places to go and people to see.

When they got down to the four-by-four, the back end was full of people. Larry shook his head in disbelief. "What the Hell?"

Cisco stepped in front of him, face to face. "You know that in Juarez, every vehicle is a potential taxi. These folks are all family and friends and they all need to go to the Paquime area. Some are even descendants of the Paquime Indians."

Larry chuckled and opened the cab door. An ancient woman was sitting politely in the middle spot, seat belt buckled. She wore a dark dress and a muted colored shall. For some unknown reason, she squealed with toothless delight when Larry started the motor. Cisco climbed in .

"Gracias, Señor Sully, these people will be in your debt." The kid sounded genuine, but Larry doubted that he would see any of these people again.

Paquimè is a historical place with a maze of ruins left by a tribe of Native Americans that have been long gone. It is a few kilometers south of Juarez and Larry enjoyed seeing some new country. He pulled the big pickup in next to a tour bus, near the ruins. The people in the pickup bed climbed out and came to him one by one saying nice things to him in Spanish or their native tongue. Larry didn't understand all the words. But the meaning was understood. He felt like some sort of a Godfather. He smiled a lot and said "de nada" to them all. The last of the group, a man who wore a straw hat that had been sprayed with blue paint around the edges, took Larry's hand and looked him in the eye for an un-comfortable amount of time. Finally he smiled and said 'we will meet again my friend', then hurried away to catch up with the others.

"You must be the new gringo in town, eh?" Ricardo was sitting up on the back of the seat of a 1963 Stingray Corvette. "I hear you want to see me."

Cisco answered for Larry. "Buenos tardes, Ricardo. This is Señor Sully. He wants to do some business and I thought you might be able to help."

Ricardo was well dressed in expensive slacks, a satin shirt that was opened to the waist to show his gold chains. Snakeskin boots completed the outfit. "Welcome to my office, Señor. I hope you understand that this is a paid consultation?"

Larry pulled out three fifty dollar bills, the predetermined amount of cash, and handed it to Ricardo. "For you, good American dollars. What I'm looking for is some not so good American dollars. I mean to buy a large amount."

"This is a very nice ride you have here, gringo," Ricardo said as he walked around the silver truck. "I will trade my classic 'Vette for it, straight across."

Larry new this was just a stall so that Ricardo could form an opinion of him. "You have a beautiful car, also." Larry walked around the corvette. It had a beautiful pearl white paint job and custom upholstery. The tires were the odd looking low profile racing tires mounted on custom spider wheels.

"Yes, very nice indeed. Such a car would make a man famous in the state of Chihuahua. Especially if he can keep it away from los banditos. Too bad that the pickup is worth so much more. I would be tempted." Larry established that he was no fool and he had made a respectful challenge.

"No one touches my automobiles," Ricardo puffed out his chest.

Larry bit back a laugh. "As it should be, Señor."

"I can get you a meeting with Don Alonso Garcia. He does business at the bull fights on Sunday at the Plaza Monumental Bullring. Just show up dressed like you are now. I will make arrangements and they will be waiting for you. His private box is above the tunnel where the bulls enter the ring. Don't worry, they'll find you when it is your turn."

"Gracias Señor, thank you. I will speak highly of you to Don Alonso," Larry was relieved this meeting was over. As he started to turn away, Ricardo reached behind him and pulled a flask.

"Have drink with me Señor Sully." It was a challenge, not a question. Larry was caught off guard. Just when he realized that he was hesitating too long, Ciscos' hand appeared on the flask.

"The gringo has a bad liver, but I would like to drink with you. To Maria, with respect." Cisco took a long pull on the bottle and handed it back to Ricardo.

"Si, to Maria," Ricardo's' sarcastic tone turned Ciscos' toast into a joke.

On the road back to Juarez, Cisco explained that Don Alonso Garcia was one of the bosses of Groupa Diablo. Most of the young gangs on the boarder were controlled by older men, just like small versions of the Mafia in the US. If Sully could establish credibility with this man, the Italian may be the next step. A meeting with Don Alonso was not about paying money. It was about respect and tradition. With important Latin men, you must show respect first, then let them know how macho you are, stopping the game just short of winning. This allowed them to keep their machismo in tact. They only way to do good business with them, is to be strong but respectful. Only then will they trust you enough to give you a real deal, not a wild goose chase.

Larry started to say something, then hesitated. Cisco picked up the cue. "Listen, Larry. My uncle told me that you were in that no alcohol program with him. He said it was very important that you don't drink. I hope you didn't think I was outta line back there, grabbing the bottle and all."

"I owe you for that one Cisco. You were perfect. I have a lot to get used to, and you helped me out of a jam that time." He wanted to tell him that he was almost more afraid of blowing his sobriety than of blowing his cover. He held his tongue, not wanting to appear weak in front of his helper. Latinos do not respect weakness.

As he tilted his head back, the evening sun filled his eyes for a quick second. The flask felt cool in his hand. The liquid was rum, Larry's' favorite, Baccardi Light. The first taste warmed his mouth and tickled his throat. As he poured more into his mouth and it went down, he felt that good burning sensation in his chest, moving to his stomach. As his head came back level, Larry was looking into a barrel of chromed steel. In that instant he could see three vivid images-the finger pulling the trigger back, the cylinder of the 357 magnum beginning to turn and the face of Bumper Blue, laughing. They were all laughing. Bumper, Ricardo, Cisco, Fast Eddie, Bob, the red headed T-man and Captain Moffitt. They were all there. And one of the day glow creatures was there, too. The creature had a slimy arm around Jackie. She was crying. Then all at once there was a bright light and a loud bang.

Larry bolted upright in bed. Sweat running between his eyebrows and a scream in his chest that would not come out. Across from the bed, a hotel mirror showed a tortured soul exhibited on his face. He fumbled with his watch. It was five nineteen. He told himself to take deep breaths, but it took several minutes for the shaking to stop. Larry had heard of "drinking dreams", but this was the first time he had experienced one.

"God, I need a drink!" he said out-loud. "No that's the wrong prayer, stupid."

Larry rolled out of bed onto his knees. "God, I'm willing, that you have all of me, good and bad. I pray that you now remove from me, my character defects which stand between me and a sober life. Grant me the strength and show me the way to do your bidding today. Amen." The compulsion past.

After washing his face with cold water, Larry rummaged through his shaving kit, the same one that used to hold those little bottles of emergency booze, and found a scrap of paper that he had tore from the list Trevor had given him. It had Trevor's' phone number on written on it. He dialed for an outside line, then the number on the scrap.

"Trevor? This is, uh, this is uh, Tom Sullivan. I was wondering if we could get together."

"Sully! It's great to hear from you. Are you just hurting or is it too late for that?"

Trevor's' voice reassured Larry. Yes there is a God. "I'm okay, but I had this dream and..."

Trevor cut him off. "Say no more, my friend. I'll pick you up in front of your hotel in ten minutes. You can wait ten minutes before you do anything stupid, can't you?"

Logic crept into Larry's' brain. "Sure, ten minutes." The phone went dead.

In the elevator it occurred to Larry that he had called a USA number to reach Trevor, who said he would be here in ten minutes. If he showed up in ten minutes he would have to be in Mexico already. Secondly, how did he know where to pick Larry up? It could be explained by all these new telephone systems, and he did see Trevor in the hotel coffee shop a couple of days ago. Larry decided to let all that go for the time being. Sobriety was his current concern. Just as Larry stepped through the hotel doors, Trevor drove up. It was thirty-one minutes past five.

"The dream was so real at first. When I woke up it seemed like a memory. I really thought for a few seconds that I had taken that drink," Larry's voice was full of excitement. Trevor had driven them across the river to Denny's restaurant in El Paso.

Waiting for the waitress to finish pouring the coffee, Trevor slumped back into the seat with that look of concern that old-timer sponsors have. The pleasant girl finally left the table. "Scary stuff, isn't it? I had dreams like that for years. You did the right thing by calling me."

Larry tried to calm himself. "You know, I've done an occasional scary thing or two in my life. That dream was the worst fear I've ever felt."

"Fear can be a good thing, Larry. A lot of positive things can come from fear." Trevor took a long drink of coffee. "It's usually the starting point for better things to come."

The simple logic of what Trevor was saying had a big calming effect on Larry. "I guess I can see that. Sounds logical."

"Let me ask you, what was the first action you took after the dream woke you?"

Larry almost giggled because he got it. "I prayed. Very sincerely I might add."

A knowing smile slid onto Trevor's face. "They say that the foundation stone for freedom of fear, is faith. Living in fear can bring evil and destruction into your life. Belief in your concept of a higher power can overcome the evil side of fear."

"So what can I do to keep from having those kind of dreams?" Larry held the coffee cup so that it warmed his hands.

"Oh, you can't stop the dreams, only make peace with them. If you did a lot of black out drinking, like I did, there will probably be more bad dreams on the way. It has to do with synaptic connections in the brain being restored, or something like that. I don't go in for all that technical stuff." Trevor flirted with the waitress while she poured another round of coffee. "Next time you will remember that you did all the right things this time. You prayed and you called me, and most importantly, you didn't have a drink."

"My sponsor told me that low self esteem and self loathing created unreasonable fear. He said that unreasonable fear will fester and grow until it consumes a persons soul." Larry was surprised at himself for sounding so profound.

Trevor added to Larry's statement. "And the antidote for unreasonable fear is a spiritual awakening Every sober alcoholic has fears and bad dreams, but you can start your day over as many times as you need to. You can also have as many spiritual awakenings as it takes to stay sober."

Larry was genuinely appreciative of Trevor's help. "I'm sure glad you were here for me this morning, T."

"Yeah, lucky thing that I was at my girlfriends house, just a few blocks away. I'd just gotten up when the phone rang. Isn't this high tech world great? That call for-warding thingy works like a charm." Trevor had answered Larry's doubts about being in Mexico almost too easily.

Shortly after Larry returned to the hotel, Cisco came by to say that he was going to Chihuahua for a couple of days to check on Fast Eddy's uncle, the gardener. Larry asked to go with him but Cisco said it would be better to wait and that his uncle's uncle may have some useful information for them.

Realizing that he sort of had a few days off, Larry drove up to Las Cruces and shot a few rounds at the shooting range at Ralph's Guns. After a late lunch he drove out to the view point above White Sands Missile Range. The view point sits in the saddle like pass over the San Andres mountains. Spreading out below to the east is the White Sands desert and in the distance, Sierra Blanca, the tallest mountain in the area, rises out of the desert floor like a majestic crown of the desert.

Larry sat on the tailgate and drank coffee out of a thermos. He remembered how he used to drive out in the country to think and drink, and later in his addiction, just to drink It was good to be alone with his thoughts for a few hours. The more he relaxed, the more he thought of Jackie. Jackie had a long neck and a pleasing line to her jaw. Remembering her put a smile on his face and a warm fuzzy feeling in his heart. He prayed that this operation would not last too long. He wanted to get back to his new, sober life.

For diner he went back to the restaurant at the City Center Motel in Las Cruces. Afterwards he attended the AA meeting in the banquet room. Trevor was there and said hello, but he was involved with an apparent new-comer. Larry enjoyed the AA meeting, but didn't share. It seemed like the easiest way to avoid complications. He then drove back to his hotel in Juarez and got a very sound nights sleep.

Cisco took a bus to Ciudad Chihuahua arriving in the early evening. He made his way on foot to his great uncles place, sort of an apartment located in a back-street ally. The tiny dwelling had a small door and one window. The thick adobe walls were over three hundred years old. Uncle Pedro's place had a main room with kitchenette in one corner and an old leather sofa in the opposite corner. A simple wooden table with homemade chairs and a hand-carved rocker completed the furnishings. In the bedroom stood an antique cannonball bed, a wedding gift from his employer back when the Flores family still controlled the hacienda on the hill. Pedro had been the gardener there for fifty-two years. Thirty years ago, the small closet had been made into a bathroom with the addition of an old water closet toilet, the type with the tank that was high on the wall. Cisco had spent teenage summers with uncle Pedro, helping with the gardening.

The craggy old man opened the door on the first knock, having just arrived home himself. Although he was only sixty-five, Pedro had an older look about him. His weathered face and stooped shoulders gave him that anonymous 'old man' look that so many hard working men adopt later in life.

"Buenos tardes uncle Pedro, are you surprised to see me?" Ciscos face was a welcome sight.

"Francisco, my favorite nephew. God has answered my prayers!"

Cisco always brought the old man gifts. A Mexican custom of respect. "Look uncle I've brought you two pair of your favorite wrangler vaqueros."

Pedro's happy face filled with pride and his eyes filled with tears.

"This is the best day in a long time, Francisco. Por favor, sit down, we have much to talk about, you and me."

"Have you eaten? Cisco said. "Let me take you down to the cantina. We can have some of Mama Flora's pollo a la chilindron. And maybe a cerveza or two."

From a table in the back, Mama Flora's Cantina looked like a scene from a spaghetti western. Cisco and Pedro ordered dinner and beer. After the usual family small talk, Cisco moved the conversation to the reason for his visit.

"So, uncle Pedro, tell me how you really are. We are all worried about you."

"Francisco, I've told you before to just call me Pedro. You are a man now." Pedro's tone was kindly scornful. "Life for me in Chihuahua has changed."

"Is it the Italians or are you missing aunt Esperanza?" Cisco showed his concern. The old mans wife had died two years before.

"I'm sure that it is both, but these people who stole the hacienda from the Flores family, are evil pigs." Pedro looked down at his plate. As a gardener, he was taught never to be judgmental. "The things that go on there now, are the work of the devil."

"Why do you stay?" Cisco knew why.

"Tradition, I suppose, what else is an old man to do. It's all I've ever done since I was thirteen years old." Pedro's eyes showed both pride and desperation.

"Do they treat you well, uncle? Do they still pay you enough to live on.?"

Pedro made a small laugh, the kind that tells it's own story. "Francisco, I'm not sure they know I exist. I work everyday except for Sunday. Everyday I go to the kitchen door and the house staff gives me a plate of food. I take home some vegetables from the garden, as I always have, only now I sell them to make ends meet. The Italians have never paid me any money. I'm not too proud to ask, but I'm too scared to ask. Everyone is scared up there."

"Have they hurt you?" Cisco was becoming more concerned by the minute.

"No. Like I said, they don't know me. I think I'm just a fixture to them, like a plant or a statue."

Cisco laughed. "Pedro, even at your age, you still move faster than a statue."

"I stay because of la familia de Flores. They are being held as slaves in their own house. The white devil with the red hair has already killed Raul and Juan, the two young men of the family. All the women in the family have been raped and tortured and are being made to serve as housekeepers and cooks. Don Roberto de Flores died of a heart-attack, while tied to a chair, watching his wife being beaten and raped. They bring whores from the city and do awful things to them. The leader, El Cigarro, is drunk all the time. The pigs with the guns do anything they want when he is not looking. And Bruno, the big foreman, is the worst of the bunch."

"God in heaven, uncle. You must not go back to that place." Cisco slammed his Corona bottle down harder than he meant to, causing other patrons to look their way.

"No, I go back so someone will know what happened to the Flores family. They have been a respected family in this valley for two hundred years. I can't let them disappear without even a whimper. I owe them my whole life, but what can an old man do. I went to the authorities. The police had been paid by the Italians and just laughed at me."

"Listen Pedro, I'm working with a man who is going to fix this for you. He will come here soon, and all this will be over. I promise you. Can you help us to help you and the Flores?"

A light shone in the old mans face. "I will do anything to help the Flores. Anything."

Cisco went on to tell Pedro of the information that Larry needed. Some of it, Pedro couldn't possibly know, and some of it he knew already. Cisco also asked for all the details it would take to plan a raid on the hacienda. In the morning, after Pedro had left for work, Cisco walked down to the market and paid two boys to help carry a large amount of groceries and necessities back to the tiny apartment. He was sure to include several items that Pedro could sell, as Pedro was far too proud to accept money. In the afternoon, he caught a bus back to Juarez.

Upon his return, Cisco went straight to Larry's Room and told him all that he had found out in Ciudad Chihuahua. Friday and Saturday, Cisco and Larry spent their time cruising through the bars and pool halls in Juarez, talking to low-life's and picking up additional information about the men at the hacienda de Flores. It seems that Al Bennette had at least twenty two men outside and nine on the inside, including Bruno, for a total of thirty-one hired guns. The Irishman and two others were mercenaries and were in charge of the grounds. Bruno and two more Italians were Mafia from Chicago and controlled the inside of the hacienda. The rest were just bandits and thugs, all known as murderers in the state of Chihuahua.

Roaming through the bars, Larry ordered cola to drink, when it seemed necessary, and nothing at all most of the time. During Saturdays' dinner in a nice hotel restaurant, Cisco opened a conversation about alcoholics.

"Señor Sully, can I ask you some questions about your drinking?"

Larry welcomed the conversation. "Sure Cisco, what's on your mind?"

"Is it hard for you to go to all these bars and not drink? Doesn't it bother you to see all these people having fun?"

"Sometimes I think about it, but I try not to. I have to see and think about things differently than I use to. To be honest with you, I'm not sure how, exactly, that it works. I think that maybe God is helping me today." Larry was too far into explaining his thoughts to turn back. "I haven't been sober for even a year, but this stuff that I learned in Alcoholics Anonymous is working overtime on me. I have a sponsor, that's a sort of a guide who teaches you stuff about alcohol, anyway, he kept saying that 'assuming we are spiritually fit, we can do all sorts of things alcoholics shouldn't do. Except, take a drink.' He also said that if we aren't ready to meet any situation where alcohol is a factor, then we still have an alcoholic mind."

"Okay," Cisco said, "but don't you feel pressured by all the people drinking and having a good time?"

"Sure, I notice. I say a lot of prayers to myself. I try to look for the bad examples in the bars. If you look closely, not that many people are really having a good time. I try to remember that it's not fun to throw up or to wake up and not remember what happened the night before." Larry took a deep breath, his hands were shaking just talking about it. "AA taught me not to live in fear. I try to live one day at a time, and if that's not working, one hour at a time or one minute at a time."

"It must take a brave man to do this, Señor Sully."

"I don't know about that, Cisco, maybe you should go ask your uncle Eddie about that. He has been sober a lot longer than I have." Larry went on to change the subject by asking about Pedro. He had had enough nervous energy spent on this alcoholic conversation. It was the first time he really tried to explain it to someone outside the program. He noticed that he had been feeling more and more, the compulsion to drink as the day went on, and that after this conversation with Cisco, the compulsion was gone. Like a big rock had been taken off his back.

Sunday morning, Larry dressed and said a very sincere prayer. Then he went with Cisco to the catholic church. They sat in the back, Cisco doing all the catholic ritual things and Larry as an observer. His father had been a Catholic, but his mother was a Methodist who really believed more in the old Native American ways of spirituality. Larry hadn't been inside any church in many years. He sat, drinking in the spiritual ambiance, and thought mostly about his own personal contact with God. A few silent prayers seemed to be appropriate for the setting.

After church, Larry and Cisco headed for the bull fights at Plaza Monumental Bullring. Located only one block from the Rio Grande Mall, on Paseo Triunfo de la Republica, it is one of over two hundred active bull rings in Mexico. The ceremonies were just starting as they arrived.

Standing in the isle, the metal frames of Larry's chrome sun glasses were becoming uncomfortably hot in the early afternoon sun. Cisco motioned to the right side of the arena.

"All the important people will be over there in the shade." As they moved around the ring, Cisco continued. "People with money and power can buy comfort, Señor Sully. Besides, it is the best place to watch the bullfight. Have you been to a bullfight before?"

"Yes, I've been twice before." Reaching the shade, Larry leaned against the outer wall in the top row. The torero was making passes at a bull. Testing his will against the bulls. "I always root for the winner."

"You mean the torero." Cisco grinned. "A great torero kills the bull with much grace."

"This is true, Cisco, but the real winner is the bull. He gets to die with honor while showing his best machismo."

Cisco conceded. "I think you understand more about our people than I thought."

They watched as the fight unfolded in the ring. The picadors rode in on their horses, sticking the bull, an auburn colored Mexican longhorn, with their decorated lances. Under the direction of the torero, his assistant planted three pairs of banderillas into the hump on the bulls back. Then it was time for the torero to take the bull. He entered the ring proud and erect, in a beautiful hand sewn costume of blue and gold. A veteran of many fights, the proud man played with the bull for a full twelve minutes before obtaining permission from the crowd to kill the bull. He played the crowd as an expert showman, teasing the bull, but making the kill easily within the sixteen minute time limit. As the crowd of tourist and locals stood and cheered, a mountain with dark sunglasses appeared in front of Larry.

"Habla Espanol, Señor Sully?" The mountain spoke with an unusually deep voice.

"Yes, ah, si. Yo habla." Larry's Spanish was not perfect but understandable.

"Don Alonso Garcia requires your company." The mountain spoke perfect English this time. "Don Alonso may speak to you in English or Espanol, but you may only answer him in Spanish, comprende, señor?"

"What about my friend, my guide?"

The mountain removed his sunglasses and looked Cisco dead in the eyes for at least an eternity. "Si, I know this one, he may come but is not allowed to speak." He held out a massive paw to show the way. Larry and Cisco moved down the steps to a box section where two more huge thugs carried MAC-10 machine pistols under their shirts. In front of the thugs were two men, both about fifty, one was very overweight, maybe five hundred pounds.

The thinner man spoke in English with a heavy accent. "Please sit here between us, Señor Sully." Larry took the vacant chair. Cisco stood to the side like a servant. "I am Alonso Garcia, and this is my friend Ivan Kosov."

"Mucho gusto, Señors." Larry noticed for the first time that the fat man with a Russian name was a well suntanned European.

"It was told to me that you wish to purchase a large amount of gringo dollars. Is that true?"

"Si, Señor," Larry felt like he was an actor in a bad movie.

"Why do you wish to do such a thing? Why do you come to me with this matter?" The man was all business.

Larry used his Spanish to explain that he was looking for an ongoing supplier to fill the needs of several clients in the United States. He told Don Alonso that he would not deal with petty street criminals on such a matter, and that only a man of Don Alonzo's stature could insure such a deal. Don Alonso appeared to be considering carefully every word. When he spoke it was with an offer.

"Señor Sully, you may have a sample of fifty thousand American dollars for fifty cents on the dollar. You must have the money by this evening."

Larry would have counter offered even if the deal was good, which it was not. It's a point of honor not to be cheated in this country. "I will consider twenty thousand at twenty-five cents on the dollar, paid tomorrow at noon."

Don Alonso grinned and turned to the fat man, who nodded as if some secret code had been passed. "Twenty five thousand at thirty cents. That is my final offer."

Larry deliberately and slowly looked from one man to the other and back again, then replied in English for the first time. "We have deal for noon tomorrow, have your man meet me at the old Guadalupe Mission. Use a paper shopping bag."

The Russian removed his small round glasses and cleaned the dust with a fresh linen handkerchief. Then nodded.

"Don Alonso, this is acceptable," he said, returning his glasses to a puffy face. "How long will you need to make a determination. I assume you will need time to get approval from your clients."

Larry replied, this time in Spanish. "A week maybe two. If they like the samples, I would like regular deliveries of at least one hundred thousand a week. Can you arrange that for me, Don Alonso?"

The Russian spoke again without looking at Larry. "Anything is possible in business of this type. Just be sure that you can deliver your end."

The mountainous bodyguard showed up. The meeting was over. The bodyguard gripped Larry's arm, inflicting much pain just above the elbow and half dragged Larry up the steps. Cisco followed.

"You were disrespectful to Don Alonso by speaking your gringo trash." The bodyguard continued to hold Larry's arm at the top of the stairs. Larry had a vision of the man throwing him over the top railing.

"I just wanted to make sure the other man understood me, too," Larry said while trying to compose himself.

"Your meeting was with Don Alonso, not El Gordo." The mountain released his grip. "Leave now and meet me tomorrow. Don't be late and be sure the money is right or we can reach out and touch several of your friends." The huge man turned and looked directly at Cisco.

Larry fought back the compulsion to rub his sore arm as he and Cisco made their way out of the arena.

"You did very well, Señor Sully," Cisco seemed happier than normal. "Do you realize what just happened? You just had a meeting with Don Alonso and El Gordo at the same time. The head of the Groupa Diablo and the biggest money man in all of Ciudad Juarez."

"Do you mean the biggest in size or business?" Larry quipped.

"This will save us much time in the future." Cisco stopped at the silver pickup.

"Let's drive over to El Paso. I need to make some secure phone calls. I'll buy you a burger at Fast Eddies." Larry and Cisco climbed in and drove off just as Trevor exited the bull ring munching on a bag of popcorn. Smiling behind chrome sunglasses, sure that he hadn't been noticed by the eager pair.

CHAPTER 7: RUIDOSO

Larry met the large guard an exchanged shopping bags of cash as planned. To make his cover story work, he had to leave town for a few days. He arranged to leave the money in a bus locker in Las Cruces so that Jerry Smith, the red headed agent, could have it checked. Part of the operation was to make sure that it was the correct counterfeit cash that they were looking for. After putting the cash in the locker, he left the key with the swing shift janitor at the bus station who also happened to be an operative of Fast Eddie's. As far as the red head knew, Larry gave the guy a few bucks to hold the key. Then it was time to get out of the area for a while.

A 'Ski Ruidoso' brochure caught Larry's eye as it lay discarded on a bench. That was a good idea. It was late summer, so the ski area was of course closed, however, Ruidoso was far enough away and had it's own Indian gaming casino. That would fit into his cover story as a place he might take the phony money to have it checked out.

The trip to Ruidoso, New Mexico was about a two and a half hour drive from Las Cruces. The route took Larry over the mountains, across White Sands Missile Range, through the towns of Alamogordo and Tularosa and across the Mescalero Apache Indian Reservation. Just out of Ruidoso on the tip of the reservation, is Inn of the Mountain Gods, a large resort owned by the tribe complete with golf course, casino, night club, several restaurants and a hotel. Larry checked in to an upscale room using one of Tom Sullivan's credit cards. He doubted very much that anyone had followed him and no one knew of his plans as it was an instantaneous decision. He figured that if he was going to hang out somewhere, this is the kind of place where Sully would stay.

Sitting in the main restaurant after a late steak dinner, he pondered his free time. There was some planning to do. He needed to check out the casino to try to get a better feel for what Tom Sullivan knew. He could go play some golf, although he hadn't done that in about eight years. Then there was the town of Ruidoso with it's quaint gift shops and tourist atmosphere, it would take some time to see the sights. The events flyer in the room had an article about the horse races at Ruidoso Downs. This was the peak of the horse racing season and it would be fun to spend a day at the races. Filling his time wouldn't be too hard. He had been to Ruidoso before and knew that a lot of drinking went on here, but he felt pretty safe. And there had to be an AA meeting somewhere around here.

As he sipped his coffee, he looked around the dinning room. Couples in various stages of relationships were all around him. A lot of them seemed to be in love. Larry suddenly had an acute attack of loneliness. The blues washed over him like an ocean wave. He had to get up and leave the restaurant for the fear that others would suddenly know how he felt. After charging the bill to his room number, he continued outside to one of the decks that overlooked the golf course and manmade lake. The memory of Jackie and their one real date together warmed him against the cool mountain air. The compulsion to call her was almost overwhelming. He stood there and argued with himself for several minutes. It was against the rules to involve her in his undercover life, however, he rationalized that he was on sort of a vacation for a few days and not really involved in the operation. After a justifiable amount of vacillation, he made a decision to call her. What damage could a phone call do, after all, no one knew he was even here.

At a bank of pay phones in the lobby, he placed the call. After five rings, her machine picked up with her recorded message. Larry let her voice ring in his ears and forgot to say anything. Beep. He redialed.

"This is your friend Larry. How are you 'double L'? Give me a call as soon as you get this. I don't care what time it is, I just really wanna talk to you." He added the phone number to the resort and his room extension.

On the way to the room, he chose a root beer and a chocolate bar from the vending machines. Maybe there was a good movie on TV. It had been years since he had watched TV with any interest. Tonight was no different, a hundred or so channels and nothing to watch. He settled for a documentary about African animals, turned the sound off, laid back on the pillows and just starred at the set.

The ringing of the bedside phone startled him awake. Larry's confusion was absolute for about ten seconds, then his mind focused and he knew where he was. He picked up the phone and looked at his watch simultaneously.

"Larry? Are you there? This is Jackie returning your call."

"Hi there, 'Double L'!" His voice was scratchy from sleep so he took a drink of dead root beer.

"Did I wake you? I'm sorry, but your message said anytime and I just got home from work," she sounded excited.

"No.....I don't know.....maybe I dosed off. Thanks for calling." He looked at the TV and saw that an aging starlet was trying to sell a group of women some sort of face cream. He picked up the remote and clicked the off button.

"The switch board answered, 'Inn of the Mountain Gods'. That's quite a name. Where is that, I mean where are you, or should I not ask that?"

Time of truth, he couldn't just lie to her. "I guess it doesn't matter, you could find out just by asking around anyway. It's a resort near Ruidoso, do you know where that is?"

"Sort of. I've never been there, but I've heard of Ruidoso. Isn't that the place in the mountains where they have the horse races?"

"Yeah, that's the place, but don't tell anyone that I'm here. Okay?"

"No I won't. God, it's great to hear from you. It's been way too long, I miss you mister mysterious."

"Me too. You know I'm working and it's not smart to make these kind of personal contacts, but I was thinking about our date and all the good friendship we built up before that. We're still friends aren't we?"

"Of course we are, and I think maybe a bit more than that, now. You know, I think you are the most special man I've met in a long time."

Larry flushed on his end of the phone. He suddenly felt more alone than he had ever been in his life. "Listen, Jackie, I have a few days off, from my work that is, and I was wondering if we could see each other."

"Sure, I'd love to see you. Can you come to town?"

"No, I can't go back to Albuquerque right now. I know this is kind of forward, but, could you come down here? I can get you your own room and I promise to be a gentleman. I just need to see you." Larry wasn't used to feeling any kind of emotional need. He felt foolish after showing this kind of weakness so easily, but waited for her response.

Jackie held the phone to her chest for a few seconds, letting her excitement fade enough to regain her power of speech, then realized that he could probably hear how fast her heart was beating, or at least that's the way it seemed.

"Well, tomorrow is my day off and I could extend it if I needed to. I have enough overtime in to choke a payroll clerk."

"Is that a yes?"

"Uh-huh, what do you want me to do? I mean, how should I get there."

He had done it now. It was too late to turn back, but it felt right to him. Damn the rules, full steam ahead.

"The brochure here in the room says that there's a daily shuttle flight from Albuquerque that leaves at ten-thirty every morning. If you can catch that flight, I'll pick you up at the local airport."

"Do I need to wear dark glasses and a wig? How about a trench coat?"

"Don't get cute. It takes years of training to do that stuff." They both laughed.

"Okay, I'll hang up now and call the airport for a ticket. Good thing big airports run twenty-four hours a day. If you don't hear right back from me, I'll see you when I get there. Good night and sleep well."

"Night. I'll be there to get you."

Larry hung up the phone and turned out the light, trying to savor every word that was spoken.

At mid-day, Larry found himself leaning against the big silver pickup, watching the commuter plane land at the airport. It taxied up to the small welcome center and off loaded the fourteen passengers and their baggage. Jackie was the last one off the plane, dressed in white jeans, a pale blue top and sunglasses. He walked out to the plane, said 'hi' and gave her a hug. She took off the sunglasses and looked him in the eyes for a few seconds, then gave a sigh, and hugged him again.

"We better get my bag, it's so good to see you!" They turned to see that her bag was already sitting alone on the baggage cart. Larry grabbed it up and they proceeded to the truck.

"Another new car?"

"It's a rental, you could call it a business car. How was your flight?"

"Oh, it was fun, I love to fly. Those puddle jumpers fly a lot lower than the big jets, so I get to see a lot more out the window. New Mexico is so pretty from the air. We flew over a lot of forest and then I could see the desert on both sides of the tree line. This part of New Mexico is like an oasis."

"You should be taking pictures. Sounds like you have a good eye for natural beauty."

"Nope, I believe in my memory, now that I have one," she chuckled at her little sobriety joke and Larry just shook his head."

On the way into town she sat close to him in the pickup, like young lovers in an old movie. Larry took it as a sign that he wasn't the only one developing strong feelings.

They decided on lunch at a café with seating on a deck reaching over the Rio Ruidoso. As they finished eating, the sun slid behind an old growth pine tree, so Jackie removed her sunglasses again. Larry loved the way she looked. Her face was kind and gentle, her dark brown hair fell softly past her long slender neck, but it was those green eyes that captivated him. He had always looked people directly in the eyes. Some found it un-nerving, not Jackie, she looked straight back with the same intensity. That moment, eye to eye, became a perfect point in time. They didn't speak. Neither one of them had the power to break the link until the waitress started to pour more ice tea.

"Penny for your thoughts?" Her voice was unruffled.

"It's just good to see you."

"You're not having one of those male obsessive fantasy's are you?"

"Why Jackie, what could you ever mean?" He said with a sly smile.

"I like you too, mystery man, but let's try and stay in the present. Okay?"

"Oh, ground rules again?"

"You know what I mean," she changed the subject. "Ruidoso is such a beautiful place. I read the chamber of commerce pamphlet on the way down here. Did you know that 'Smokey the Bear' came from around here?"

"Yeah, over near Capitan, a few miles to the north. Billy the kid hung out a few miles to the east in Lincoln, and the Roswell is about an hours drive from here. Lot's of history around here. Would you like to see some of the sights?"

"Sure, sounds like fun, but first, why don't you show me to the room you promised. I'd like to freshen up a bit."

Larry didn't take her for the 'freshening up' type, so his thought was that it must be a signal about the room arrangement. He wasn't disappointed, he had no expectations of sleeping together. He had learned that much about Jackie and would respect her decisions, as promised. He pulled a room key with a brass number plate out of his shirt pocket.

"Room 207," he said and handed her the key. "I'm in 212, almost across the hall." The look on her face told him he was correct in his assumption. One of the things he had learned in sobriety was to always do the 'right thing' even if your desires or ego said otherwise. They drove through town to the resort where he left her in her room for an hour or so, then showed her around the resort.

They skipped dinner and rented horses at the resort stables for the evening. Both had been on a horse before, but for each it was a long time ago. The trail led them into the woods along a brook and after an hour or so they stopped to rest. The stable man had given them a thermos of coffee and a blanket for their evening ride. Jackie poured the coffee and they sat quietly on a fallen tree, watching the water bubble past. They talked about the trees and the mountains, Larry felt relaxed for the first time in ages. Jackie finally turned the conversation to more personal matters.

"Can I ask you a couple things about your work?"

"There's not much to tell."

"I feel that I need to know things. I know better than to pry about specific details. I just want to know things like. Is it dangerous? Are you gone a lot? Are you happy with what you do? You know, stuff like that. A girl needs to know when she should worry and when everything is okay."

"Does this mean we're going steady?" Jackie punched his arm in response to his sarcastic tone.

"Please, Larry, you know I care about you. It's just so hard when you give me so little information."

"Well, let's see, what can I tell you? I used to be a regular officer for the Albuquerque PD, then once upon a time they needed someone to work undercover in Santa Fe, you know, to catch the bad guys. It was an FBI case and they liked what I did. Nobody has asked me to wear a uniform since."

"So you work for the city or the FBI?"

"Both, and then some. I don't even know who I really work for. They just keep loaning me out to every police organization you could think of."

"Do you mean lot's of different places?"

"Yeah, they send me all over the United States and sometimes even out of the country."

"Wow, no wonder you are so secretive. How do you keep it all straight? I mean, it must be pretty darn hard not to loose yourself in all that."

"I don't know how I do it. I used to just drink until I was anesthetized. But now it's different. It's like I can see consequences for my actions and the actions of others. And I don't just mean jail time for crimes. Somehow, for the first time in my life, I feel that there really is some sort of greater moral standard, not just the law. It's not all black and white like it used to be." He had just realized that he had expressed doubts about his continuing ability to do his job, but he didn't want to explore that with Jackie, at least not yet.

She remained quiet for a while, soaking up what Larry had said. Finally, she just had to ask the obvious.

"It really is dangerous, isn't it?" She reached out and touched his face. He welled up with emotion, it had been an eternity since anybody cared about him enough to worry for his safety. He fought back tears and cleared his throat.

"No, not really, I'm just a guy who has a talent for getting information. I leave the 'Dirty Harry' stuff for the other guys." It was sort of a lie and sort of the truth, but how could he tell her about the terror that went with the job, or the times when the back up was just a little too slow for comfort. He had already lost one woman over the job. Well, the job and the booze to be fair, but Sally had blamed a lot of their problems on the dangerous work he did. He stood and pulled her to her feet for a long hug.

"We better get back. I don't know if these rent-a-horses know their way in the dark."

After returning the horses, they took a walk through the casino and had burgers from the casino snack bar. Jackie was tired from the long day after a late shift and retired to her room around ten o'clock. Both of them had a lot to think about.

The next day Jackie and Larry spent the morning visiting the tourist shops in the village. The downtown association had spent a fortune making Ruidoso a comfortable place to spent money on quaint trinkets and expensive works of art. With two completely different tourist seasons, it is a town of much diversity. The wintertime snow- boarders and ski bunny crowd have completely different tastes than the cowboys and horse people who overrun the town during the summer. The result is a cross-breading of cultures and ideas in everything from jewelry to music to T-shirts. Another fantastic by product of the large tourist trade is the great eateries. The pair had an unbeatable Mexican food lunch and decided on the race track for the afternoon and evenings entertainment. It was great just to get to know each other a little better without getting into heavy conversations, just hanging out and enjoying each others company.

At days end they ended up in Larry's room with hot fudge Sundays from room service, a decadent treat. Jackie pushed the tasty confection away, half finished.

"Well, I got to admit it, you sure know how to show a girl a good time. How did you know that I'm a chocoholic? Chocolate's the short cut to my heart you know."

"Naw, a true chocoholic wouldn't be stopping short."

"Oh, God, I'm so full I'm gunna bust, but I really enjoyed it. In fact, I think I've had the best time of my life, being here with you. Thank you, I needed this break."

"Sounds like you've been working hard, Double L?"

"Yeah, you know I work in the trauma center and I also substitute as a flight nurse on the helicopter."

"You never told me that you flew at work."

"Only when they need an extra hand, it was just another certification at first. You know, to make more money, but then I started liking it. I did a few trips in the fixed wing medical flights, then they put me in a helicopter and I loved it."

"That sounds like fun."

"It's more than fun, it's exciting. They go where the action is. Anything big happens, you're at ground zero and the flight nurse is in charge of the scene as long as they are on the ground. Adrenaline and responsibility all wrapped up together."

"Don't us alkies try to avoid those kind of stressful situations?"

"It's what I do, I can handle it. The real stress comes from the big choices in life. The trauma department keeps hinting at me taking over a shift. I would have a team of the core people to boss around everyday. Doctors, nurses and technicians. The idea is to keep teams together so that they work more efficiently."

"I'm surprised that a nurse would have the top job. I would think they'd choose a doctor."

"No, the doctors are too important on the front lines, they need someone who can stand back and make the logistical decisions during times of crisis."

"Sounds like a good job for you, you're so level headed."

"Yeah, but, the problem is that the flight crews want me to become a full time flight nurse, and I love to fly."

"Oh, I see. I'm not the only one who thinks you're the best. Do you have to decide soon? Seems like you're kind of getting some of both right now."

"Thanks for the complement. I think it is going to come up pretty soon, but right now nobody has said anything official. It's not a money decision, both jobs pay well. The trauma job is a good career move and the flying job is an adventure."

"People say it's best to do what you love. Makes the wheel of life turn bit easier."

"Do you love what you do?"

Larry pulled up short and thought for a few seconds before answering. When he spoke his voice was almost sad.

"I guess I used too love it. Now I'm not so sure. I like doing the right thing and I do love solving the puzzles, getting the information. Investigating is fun, but the undercover thing, I just don't know anymore. I had a natural talent for it, they said. But they aren't the ones who have to go out and live among the scumbags of the world, pretending to be their friend and hoping nothing goes wrong. There was this one guy, a child molester.........." He realized he was breaking his promise to himself not to talk about certain things.

"I'm sorry, Little Lady, it's not good conversation for a date." She was so easy to talk to. He just wanted to tell her everything, but that wouldn't be fair and he thought it would probably chase her away.

"Hey, it's okay if you want to talk about it sometimes."

"No, this the time when we are suppose to put our best foot forward. It wouldn't be fair to muddy the water with a bunch of awful war stories and experiences, now would it?"

"You're such a sweet man." She was on her feet moving around the small table. "Hey, mister mysterious, I can take anything you have to tell me." She leaned down and kissed him. He stood up and embraced her with a second more powerful kiss.

"Mmm, this feels so good." He hadn't had a kiss so passionate in a very long time. It almost made his knees buckle.

She put her hands on his chest as if to push him away, but laid her head on his shoulder instead.

"Larry, I think what we're doing feels right, too. It would be very easy to let down my guard and let nature take it's course, but I think we should wait. We both need to settle some things, I think, and, well, let's just wait until you get back from your, ah job. Okay?"

"Do you think I was trying to push you into something?" He sounded truthfully concerned. "I didn't expect anything when I asked you to come here."

"No, no. You have been a perfect gentleman, just like you promised. I just want us to take our time with this relationship and take positive action towards each other instead of just reacting to our feelings and environment. Does that make any sense?"

"Sounds pretty profound there, Little Lady." More bogus John Wayne. "I just aim to please, mam."

Jackie grabbed both of his hands and stepped back to face him with a questioning smile. He understood her need to be put at ease.

"Really, it's okay with me, too. You aren't alone in wanting to be cautious. You know I haven't exactly been good at this sort of thing in the past, and you are right, I do have sort of a lot going on right now. This work assignment is going to be a test on my program, that's for sure."

"How are you holding up?"

"Fine, so far. There is this guy.....well I'd better not say. Anyway, I feel strong and I'm trying to stay focused."

"Use the phone if you can, if you're in need that is. You should call your sponsor or you can call me if you want. Isn't Bob your sponsor? Bob, the car dealer?"

"Yes, Bob, but it's not okay with what I'm involved in right now. I stretched the rules just about as far as I could by calling you, and I'm not even working anywhere close to here. I think I'll be okay, though."

"Well, you better be, 'cause I want you back in one piece. You understand me, Mystery Man?"

They shared another long kiss and embrace, after which, she pushed him away gently.

"NEWS FLASH! NURSE EXPLODES INTO FIRE WHILE ON VACATION! MYSTERY MAN SOUGHT FOR QUESTIONING! I think I'd better return to my room now. I need to calm down for my flight back tomorrow."

"Oh, you're not going to leave already, are you?"

"Now don't whine. Duty calls, and we probably both need to get back to work. How long are you going to be gone."

"Don't know. We'll just have to see. These cases take a little time, and to rush it could be...ah... irresponsible," Larry tried hard to not make it sound dangerous. He also realized that she had reached her current boundary for this relationship. He wasn't unhappy about it at all, in fact everything was perfect in his world, with the one exception that he had to return to Mexico and the case at hand.

The next morning they had brunch on the patio and he took her to meet the shuttle plane. The week had gone well. He had never even had to tell her that she was checked in under an assumed name or that he was now know as Sully. It just never came up. It seemed to him that the universe was in sink and the future looked bright. That night and the next one he investigated the local Indian gaming casino, amassing as much background information as his brain could hold, just in case. Then he drove back to Ciudad Juarez, feeling refreshed and confident.

CHAPTER 8: THE ITALIAN

The Flores family came to the Americas by ship in 1782. Don Juan Sancho de Flores was a mining engineer, commissioned by the crown, to develop gold and silver interests in the recently founded Ciudad de Chihuahua. Although Don Sancho had very little knowledge of precious metals, he had lots of advisors from the church. His family had been the excavators of many of the great public and religious buildings in Spain. With his wife, Esmerelda, who came to the new world five years later, the Flores family flourished with four strong sons, and thirteen grandsons. By the eighteen hundred and forties, Hacienda de Flores stood on a hill overlooking the city full of family, friends and servants. A true pillar of the community where a large number of social affairs took place each year. During the next sixty years, Mexico suffered many small battles, revolutions, take-overs and diseases. The family Flores lost more of their young men than most households. At the turn of the twentieth century Don Paco Sancho de Flores stood with his young wife Christina and only the family name to rebuild the empire the Flores family once commanded. Obtaining a lifetime contract to supply the Mexican army with beef and horses, granted mostly out of respect for the family name, the young Don Sancho hired Indians to catch wild horses, half of which he sold to start his herd of Mexican longhorns. By the time he turned the family holdings over to Don Roberto in nineteen forty-four, the Flores name was flush with new fortune from re-acquiring the mining interests that proved profitable during both the Spanish revolution and World War II. He had also hired a young Indian boy named Pedro, to help in the vast gardens that supplied the Hacienda with all matter of food and natural beauty.

Young Pedro learned fast and became the boss of the grounds at the age of twenty-two. For the next twenty years he commanded a team of over thirty subordinates who were so proficient that the Flores became known in Ciudad Chihuahua for their charitable donations of fresh food to the needy. In the nineteen seventies, much modernization came to the Hacienda and the need for large truck gardens diminished. The gardeners' work crew dwindled to five or six people and Pedro took more work onto himself than ever before. Grass and flowers were more important to the new generation than good fresh food. When the Italians came to the Hacienda, the remaining outdoor crew fled back into the city never to return. Only Pedro remained tending to the flowers and a small garden. Mowing the grass on a riding mower, never making eye contact with the new rulers of Hacienda de Flores. For some unknown reason, they left him alone to do his work. Allowing him to leave daily when everyone else, the family, the servants and the stable hands were held hostage or killed. To some people, old men just become invisible.

Pedro had many thoughts of revenge and retribution, burning down the house, poisoning the food or water, killing the livestock and he even entertained the idea of slitting the throat of the Italian boss, referred to as El Cigarro by the locals, while he slept his drunken sleep. Pedro didn't have the resolve at his age to carry out such ideas, but he returned every day to hope for a way to help La Familia de Flores.

Pedro knocked softly on the kitchen door. The grand-motherly figure of Rosa Lopez, who had been the hacienda cook for thirty-two years, opened the door.

"Hola Pedro," she said as a tear fell down Rosa's cheek. "This is not a good time for you to eat." She opened the door a bit wider, showing Bruno sitting at the table with one hand up the uniform skirt of Emanuella Flores, one of the remaining family members who's husband Raul, Bruno had already killed. With his other hand he was tipping back a bottle of whiskey. Bruno's back was to Pedro. Pedro looked deliberately down at the sharp grass trimmers in his hand. Rosa understood the look and shook her head no as she reached out and touched Pedro's hand. "It's not worth it my old friend."

Pedro made more silent vows as he backed away and turned. Glancing back at Rosa he said, "lo siento, Rosa. I'm a sorry old man but help is coming." Rosa closed the back door.

In the kitchen the tension was overwhelming. Emanuella was not a willing partner for Bruno's advances, although Bruno had had his way with her a dozen times before; the first time as her husband lay dying in the stable. Bruno pulled her onto his lap by her long silky hair and ripped open her uniform exposing her round breasts that bore the scares of Al Bennette's cigar. Her face showed no emotion. The dead face of those who have been pushed past their natural level of endurance. Rosa picked up the shallow basket she used to carry food and went into the large pantry. She sat on a sack of potatoes and cried as Bruno shoved Emanuella onto the table and began his grunting.

In the grand room, although it was after two in the afternoon, Al Bennette was just waking up from last night's stupor. Apparently, he had passed out sitting at the baby grand piano that sat in its own small alcove. His cheek showed an impression of black and white keys, his bloodshot eyes added to the colorful mask.

"Bruno!" He bellowed. "Bruno! Were the hell are you when I need you?"

In the kitchen Bruno with-drew and brushed Emanuella roughly to the floor. "Christ, that old man knows how to ruin a good thing." He deliberately stepped on Emanuella's hand, repairing his zipper as he left the kitchen.

Bennette had made it as far as an eighteenth century velvet sofa before collapsing .

"Bruno, tell that lazy cook to get my usual breakfast and pour me a drink." Al liked scrambled eggs with green peppers and cheese for breakfast.

Bruno complied, returning with a bloody-Mary.

"Sit with me Bruno. I've got something to tell you," Bennette often demanded an audience for no apparent reason.

Bruno sat. "Yes, boss. What is it."

"Son, you must know that we will be here in Chihuahua for a long time, maybe forever." Bruno hated it when he called him son. "We must think about our retirement."

"Do you think the Chicago bosses will just leave us down here?" Bruno tried to show concern even though he had resigned himself to this place long ago.

"Let me ask you something," Al's tone was so serious that he almost sounded sober. "I know that the bosses assigned you to me when I was forced to come to this wretched place. Do you still owe an allegiance to them or are you my man?"

Bruno chose to live another day. "I am your man, Al, but I swore a blood oath to the Mafia, just like you did. Are you asking me to give up that oath?"

Bennette leaned forward and lit a huge cigar, puffed twice and considered the smoke. "What I'm asking is your opinion. Do you think we should build our own little empire right here? For the benefit of us and our domain?"

It was Bruno's turn to answer slowly. "I have seen that the biggest bosses, in charge of the biggest neighborhoods, always have some enterprises of their own to pay the overhead. So to speak."

"Then you would be with me if I chose to make us both very rich?" An offer that no Mafia man could resist.

"Yes boss. You should know that I report only to you. Before we left Chicago, there was some trouble for me. It seems that a certain niece of a Don came up pregnant. The finger was pointed at me, I don't know why, but she was sixteen and I got to go on this extended trip. I have the feeling that I may not be asked to return."

Bennette felt confident. This worked well for him no matter what happened. Bruno was a perfect scapegoat if it all fell apart. And a good bodyguard in the mean time.

"Tell me about the other two Italians that you brought here."

"Okay, that's no problem. They are both cousins of mine. Like brothers. And neither of them are made men. Just soldiers from the rank and file. They think they are on a mission and that I am their general." Bruno did not want any competition for Al's favor. "The outside men are all just hired help, with no vested interest. A little money, a few senoritas and a license to kill once in a while. Simple men, really. My kinda guys, and useful."

"That's good, son. Something has come up with the German. It's far bigger than everything else we're into down here," Bennette sounded more sober all the time. "This could make us both very rich. I need you to be a very active part in the operation. More than a bodyguard. Much, much more."

Al had finally got Bruno's attention. "Well that gives you three options. Buy the European puke out, kill the bastard, or steal the plates and the process."

"How about all three, in turn, so to speak?" Al had made Bruno actually smile. They raised their glasses in an unspoken toast.

Pedro returned to the kitchen door an hour or so later, not so much for food as to check on Rosa. She had opened the door for fresh air and was busy making a pie when she noticed him in the doorway.

"Glad you're back, Pedro, I saved a plate of beans and rice for you. The pigs ate all the beef today," Rosa's attempt at cheerfulness was weak.

"I had to be sure you were all-right, Rosa."

"Oh, they have found some other perversion for distraction this evening," Rosa placed a pie in the oven and sat a plate on the table for Pedro.

"I am but a worthless old man, Rosa, but I worry so about you and the remaining women and children." Pedro realized that Rosa was offering a place at the table for him. The first time since the Italians had taken the hacienda. Lately he had taken his daily meal on the back steps.

He sat at the table and steeled his resolve. Pedro knew he could be killed for bringing this kind of attention to himself. His life the past few months had depended upon keeping in the mental shadows of the evil ones. As he took a mouthful of spicy rice, Rosa continued the conversation.

"You and I are both old, Pedro, I have no illusions about the situation here," Rosa poured herself a cup of coffee and sat down with her friend. "They will hurt us if they find out what I am about to say. Do you wish to hear it?"

Pedro nodded and placed a callused hand on Rosa's wrinkled palm. "Our lives have been good all these years working for the Hacienda de Flores. A little danger means nothing if we can help the family."

"Oh, Pedro, you are a knight in shinning armor to me. I want you to do something. It will take a plan. Maybe you will need some help," Rosa's voice was shaky. "Did I hear you say that help was coming?"

"Si, Rosa, but I don't know who or when. My nephew, Francisco, told me."

"Francisco, the young boy who helped in the garden a few years ago?" Hope had found it's way into her voice. "He must be a fine man now. You told him of our plight?"

"He came to my house to tell me that someone was working against the evil ones, and he is part of it. He needed all kinds of information," he tried to sound as confident as he could. "We just need to hold on a while. Is everyone okay."

"These men are getting worse. El Cigarro is drunk all the time now. I never leave the kitchen or servants quarters in this part of the house, except to serve the meals, but the others say he passes out two or three times a day. They have to clean up his vomit and urine. He makes the younger women bath him and, and, ...ah...," tears were flowing down Rosa's face.

"I know, they are forced to do unspeakable things," grave concern filled Pedro's speech. "Have they hurt you?"

"Women can be strong, Pedro. They have raped and beaten all of us. The Flores women and the house staff. Some have been tortured for the sadistic pleasure of Bruno and Señor Bennette. All except the children. We have managed to keep them quiet in the servants quarters and the cellar," she stopped to catch her breath in-between sobs. "That is what we need your help with. It won't be long until the children are under the cruelty that the rest of have endured. Pedro, you must help get the children out of here."

A long silence preceded Pedro's reply. "I know things about this house that probably no-one else alive knows. Maybe you heard rumors over the years of secret passageways. If you did, they are true. I'm ashamed that I have forgotten about them until now. We could get all of you out. A few each night."

"No! Only the children. If they missed anyone of us women they would start torturing and killing us," Rosa's face left no question about the truth. "You know that Juan Ricardo Roberto Flores is the last surviving male of the family. He is only nine, but he must survive to become the new Don Flores someday. To carry the family name to his own sons and reclaim the holdings of La Familia de Flores."

"As you wish, Rosa. I can get them out in a couple of days. I will arrange for someone to pick me up after work in the evening. Let me tell you where an opening is to the hidden passageways."

Pedro went on to explain how several of the different patriarchs had created and added to the hidden system for different reasons. Some of the passages had been built for escape, some for spying and some just for convenience. It was a big hacienda, looking more like a hotel on the inside than a house. Including the servants quarters, of eleven tiny rooms and a small parlor, the rooms numbered forty-two. The one hundred foot "great" room, where social functions were held, featured three lead crystal chandeliers, several large sculptures in the middle and antique furniture along the walls. With the grand staircase and connecting formal dinning room that could seat over forty for dinner, the great room was the center of the house. It was also the nearest place for the children to enter the secret passageways. Years ago, a small earthquake has closed off the opening to the servants quarters that more than one Don Flores had used as a tunnel of love. All the other entrances were in the upstairs rooms, out of reach for this purpose.

Before leaving he told Rosa exactly where the children had to be and at what time they were to be there. Then he walked home with a lighter heart, knowing that he, at last was about to take action to help the family. He had set the day for Thursday, two evenings ahead. He was sure he could enlist his former workers, who now worked at a farm father up he road, to help with a ride. They hated the

Italians also, having lost their jobs, and they had an old pickup with a covered bed.

Al Bennette stumbled into conciseness on Thursday morning about eleven o'clock. It occurred to him that he was in the process of walking across the floor when he came to. Only a chronic alcoholic could understand that feeling. Realizing that you have absolutely no control over your life, what so ever. Somewhere along the line, alcoholic behavior had replaced your intended life. At first, each day may be an adventure and you see yourself as sort of a silly drunk. Then you realize that you can't help what you do. You may know that your actions are wrong, but be powerless to stop yourself from doing them. Then a deep seated fear overcomes you. The fear of what your uncontrollable actions may do to you. Most alcoholics at this stage become extremely angry. The fear manifests itself in two ways. First the desire to get drunk and feel nothing; second, the compulsion to lash out at other people.

"Bruno, where are you man?" 'Someday that man will have to suffer for being so inattentive', Al thought.

"Right behind you boss," Bruno was coming out of the kitchen with a plate of breakfast. "Here is the food you ordered."

"Food! Who the hell can eat now?" Bennette toppled the plate onto the floor as Bruno handed it to him "Bring me a woman to shave and bath me. And get that lazy downstairs maid to clean up this mess." What he really meant was 'bring me a woman to beat and don't remind me that I was blacked out.'

"Okay boss," Bruno knew better than to contradict Al Bennette. "Isn't that German guy gunna come today?"

"Sure, sure. You an' me are gunna have a little talk 'bout it later," Bennette picked up an opened half-empty bottle of Jack Daniels from the table next to the stairs. "Now quit pushin' me and get me that whore with the nice tatas!"

Bennette took a long pull on the bottle, let out a horrible yell and climbed the stairs. The master bedroom suite had a modern Jacuzzi style bath tub big enough for two or three people. Someone had turned on the water before he got there. He stripped and stepped in complaining loudly that it was too cold. By the time Valentina, the wife of Juan Julio Flores, now deceased, arrived, Bennette had drained the bourbon bottle and called for more.

As Valentina's shaking hand poured from the new bottle into a glass, she spilled a small amount on his arm. Bennette swore and backhanded her. She dropped the bottle and it broke. As she bent over to pick up the pieces, he slugged her hard in the right temple, opening a cut above her eye with his diamond ring. She fell backward, her foot coming down hard on the broken glass for balance. A chunk of glass the size of a orange slice protruded from her foot. She tried but could not hold back the tears. The pain of the two wounds was immense. Gathering all her strength and bravery, she sat and pulled the sharp object from her foot. Before she could do anything to stop the bleeding, he grabbed her hair and pulled her back to the tub.

"Get back here you friggin' slut, get down there and do your business. You know what I want." Bennette pulled her roughly across the edge of the tub by her hair, knocking the wind from her lungs. Just as she fought to fill her lungs, he pushed her head under the water towards his crotch. Valentina inhaled but it was only water. Bennette was too drunk to realize that she was drowning. After struggling for almost a minute. She went limp.

With an evil laugh, Bennette stood up, pulling her lifeless body up by the neck, and looked into her eyes. The life had gone. "Damn it all! Someone bring me another one of the Mexican whores. This one's broken," He yelled loud enough to be heard in every room. He then shoved her limp body away from the tub and sat back down. "More booze too. Damn it you people know I ain't got all day. You friggin' Spics are always trying to screw me up."

Valentina's body fell hard against a velvet parlor chair. The jolt pushed the water from her lungs and as she fell sideways, she took a reflexive breath. Then another. She was alive. As Esmerelda climbed into the tub with Bennette, Valentina lay quietly bleeding. She stayed on the floor appearing as lifeless as she could until he had gone. Bennette never noticed.

"Stay out of sight until we know if El Cigarro thinks he has killed you or not. If he thinks you are dead, then you can go with the children," Esmerelda put a good dressing on Valentina's foot and made a compress for her head.

"I can not leave you here with these monsters. We must both go." Valentina winced.

Esmerelda tossed her head back. Fire shone in her black eyes. "I'm not as frail as you are my dear sister-in-law. I can handle these swine. My plan is to stay long enough to have a chance to kill at least one of them."

The next day Rosa got word to Pedro that El Cigarro thought he had killed Valentina. She would accompany the children when Pedro smuggled them out. Pedro made a false grave next to the real grave of Valentina's dead husband. He had dug too many graves in the hacienda's cemetery. It had been his job ever since he was sixteen to bury the dead of the Flores family. They had all died of normal causes until the Italians showed up. This year he had buried Don Roberto, Raul, Juan, Don Roberto's wife Catrina, two maids, a stable boy and the ranch foreman from Texas, a cowboy named Rex. Pedro wondered what had happened to the fine heard of cattle that the family owned. Probably rustled by neighbors. The best horses were in the barn and he kept them fed. The main body of horses wandered the property at their own pace. Eighty-two thousand acres was enough room for the horses to survive on. He stopped at Don Roberto's grave and made a vow to see the end of the evil ones.

"All will be restored Don Roberto. You have my word as a gentleman," Pedro Patted the large tombstone. "Sleep well old friend."

Dressed and smoking, Bennette paced across the floor of one of the sitting rooms. This room had all the modern stuff like computer hookup, television, stereo, video machine and control box for the satellite TV.

"This is the deal Bruno. Quit fiddling with that damn remote and listen." Bruno threw the remote on a coffee table. "We gotta pay the German for today's delivery, then we have a chance to buy his operation. He is asking three million. He'll probably take less. Once we have control of the operation, we're gunna market the money to the Chicago bosses and other fools, too. Cut out the middleman and keep all the profits from this end."

"Do you have that kind of money to pay him boss?" Bruno was more interested now than ever.

"Don't worry about it, I still got most'a my money that we came here with. You know we got this fine house for free. All because that fool Roberto asked me to dinner. Remember his face when we showed up in force the next day. Dicks hard an' guns a blazing?" Bennette stopped long enough to pour himself another drink. "That kraut bastard wants his money wired to one of those secret accounts. We know something about those kinda things, don't we son?"

"Yeah boss, the mob couldn't operate these days without computers and secret accounts," Bruno was going to enjoy this. "That bitchy bookkeeper with the blonde hair and glasses back in the states taught me all we need to know."

Bennette took a long draw on his cigar and let the smoke escape slowly. "What I had in mind was the old double transfer scam. Can you pull that off, son?"

"It's as easy as sending email, Boss. We wire money into his account, let him enter his access codes and capture them in a cache file on our computer. As soon as he's gone, we retrieve the codes and transfer the money into a third account of our choosing." Bruno smiled. "Ain't high tech a cool way to do crime. Don't even get your hands dirty."

"Well, I was plannin' on you getting a little blood on 'em," Bennette's meaning was crystal clear to Bruno, and he liked the idea.

"No problemo, boss. I'll do the bodyguard first. He thinks he's real tough," Bruno picked up a dirty wine glass. "He hasn't met me in an alley, yet." His massive fist close around the glass he was holding until it shattered. Bruno sucked blood from a minor cut and smiled sardonically.

"Yeah, that's what I'ma talkin' 'bout," Bennette pointed in the air with his cigar like it was a sword. "I wanna see that aristocratic prick cut down to size. We need ta wait a few days until we know the operation works. That's your job. All yous gotta do is oversee a bunch of dirty Mexicans and make sure they don't go ripping nothing off."

"It's a done deal, boss." Bruno crossed the room and poured himself a stiff drink, at last, he felt like there was a way to make something more of himself in this unbearable place and maybe, just maybe, he could rid himself of this dinosaur that he worked for.

Having gone through the usual tense greetings and small talk, Bennette and the German sat at the big dinning table with Carlos and Bruno leaning against opposite walls. A few chairs away the same two young girls who were at their last meeting, dressed in the same evening gowns, sat with their salads. They both looked much worse than before. Carlos was visibly angry, but controlled himself. Both girls showed bruises on their shoulders and necks, one of the evening gowns was torn. Their names were Tina and Vicki, having opted for the more American versions of their traditional Spanish names. Tina was trembling and taking short rapid breaths while twisting her napkin obsessively in her lap. Vicki was trying to eat, but a small amount of salad dressing was dribbling from the corner of her mouth. After laying her fork down as if to wipe her face with the napkin, Vicki's eyes rolled back into her head and then she passed out in her plate. The German started to get up to help her.

"Leave her alone, stay where you are!" snapped Bennette. "She just another Mexican whore that can't hold her drugs." Bennette's contempt for the locals was full of hatred for anyone he could put beneath him. He considered the Mexican people to be slow moving cockroaches, just waiting to be squashed beneath his boot.

Von Stien sat back down, but Carlos moved up and pulled her head off of the table. What happened next was very quick. Bruno started around the table as Carlos wiped her face. Bruno's movement caught Carlos' eye, but so did movement past Bruno in the next room. It was Pedro opening the secret passageway. Three small forms ran for the opening. As they disappeared inside the wall, the larger figure of Valentina appeared. To accommodate Valentina, Pedro pushed the opening wider causing a creaking sound. Everyone, heard the sound. Reacting with lightning speed, Carlos worked the slide on his M9, which as usual, he had in his right hand. With the loud metallic click of the gun, the clock stopped. It was as if a movie had been paused in a VCR. Carlos made eye contact with Pedro as he closed the opening, then Von Stein. The German had seen the dash for safety in a mirror reflecting off of the verandah glass and raised an eyebrow to signal Carlos that he understood.

The German jumped up. "Carlos, behave yourself. We are guests! Safety that gun and stand back."

Carlos finished wiping Vicki's face, leaned her against Tina, flipped the safety on the weapon and stuck it in his belt. The impromptu diversion had worked. The sound of the gun quickly replaced the sound of the secret door in everyone's mind. Bruno returned to his bodyguard stance with a scowl. No-one doubted the dangerous sincerity of Carlos's resolve. Normal time resumed at the dinner table.

After dinner, Bennette led the group into sitting room with all the modern conveniences.

"I heard from my people," he said. "The bosses are interested in buying the operation. To open the negotiations I thought you would like to get paid for today's shipment. Bruno."

Bruno produced a Halliburton case from a locked cupboard, opened it and counted out ninety thousand dollars and closed the case. Von Stein looked casually at the stack of money. No need to check it. He new they would never cheat him at this stage of the deal. He pulled out his pipe and started to pack it as if he were next to the fireplace at home in Germany.

"Well, Mr. Wolf, ain't you gonna check it? I assume you brought the shipment with you," Bennette was playing nice, so far.

The German nodded to Carlos. Carlos exited the room and reappeared with a duffel bag from the armored Mercedes, unzipped it and dumped the contents on the coffee table. A million dollars was impressive to look at, even if it was counterfeit. Bruno sat down to count and examine the cash. He tried to keep his hands from shaking. It was the first time he had ever seen so much money. Having come from a poor background, he found it hard to keep his tough guy appearance and not drool or giggle.

"What was to keep us from just taking it out of the car," Bennette asked with a smirk. "You's guys got some kind ah, huevos."

"Bomb," Carlos said softly.

"What!" Bruno said coming to his feet. Bennette stopped mid-drink, elbow in the air, afraid to move.

"Just a small bomb," Carlos said softly. The Italians had never heard him speak before. Carlos reached across the table and picked up the duffel bag and unzipped the pouch on the end. Reaching in he pulled out two sticks of dynamite with wires and some sort of electronics all duct-taped together.

"It's all-right," He said as he laid the bomb on the table next to the money. From his pants pocket he pulled a small transmitting device. He flipped a switch. A red light on the device came on. "Motion sensor, nobody gets it for free." He turned off the red light and turned on a green light. "Remote boom. Nobody touches Señor Wolfs car." He turned off the green light and tossed the control to Bruno. A gift for you. Just a toy."

Bruno picked up the control carefully and examined it. "I assume that I don't push this blue button until I'm ready. How do I disarm this thing?"

Carlos smiled. "Oh, no one can do that. It was built to be used. Just save it for, how do you Americans put it, a rainy day. Save it carefully."

Bennette poured himself another drink and laughed out loud. "Your man really had us going, Mr. Wolf. For a minute, even I thought we were all dead."

Bruno smiled. "Thanks, I'll find a use for it some day." He put the bomb and the case of money into the cupboard and pocketed the remote. Carlos bit the inside of his mouth hard to keep from laughing at Bruno's stupidity. He correctly guessed that the Italian muscle man had never heard of a 'Trojan horse'

"Now that we are through with the theatrics, have you an offer for me, Mr. Bennette?"

"Sure thing, Mr. Wolf," Bennette sat in a rocking chair as Von Stein sat on the sofa. Bennette considered himself a good poker player, but really didn't care if he won this negotiation, thinking that they would reclaim the money anyway. "How 'bout a million and a half bucks? In your account as you suggested. We have the computer link up right here."

"Sorry, Mr. Bennette, that won't do, try again," The German showed no emotion at the low offer. "I intend to retire from this crime life. So you must do better than that."

"Look my job is to get the best price for the bosses. If you have a low price in mind, tell me and maybe we can save all this pussying around," Bennette was starting to slur his words again.

"If you insist. Here is what I need to retire on. Two million for the retirement and six hundred-thousand to pay my current expenses and train your man. I assume Bruno will handle the operation for you."

"Make it two big ones and five hundred-thousand and it's a deal. And two months training."

"You have an agreement on the money, but he only needs two weeks training. Bruno doesn't need to learn to make it, just how to check it and keep the employees from stealing."

"Okay, shall we transfer the money, now?" Bennette pointed at the computer in the corner.

"Plenty of time for that. Let's get Bruno trained first." Throughout the dinner and negotiations, Von Stein remained cold and indifferent, showing the emotions and personality of a cardboard cut-out. His attitude made it clear to the Italians that he would never be one of their allies.

As the German was driven away, Bruno and Bennette proceeded to get drunk and gloat over their good fortune. Each harboring their own version of the future. Bennette wishing to be 'king of the mountain' and Bruno wishing to be rid of Bennette and out of this miserable place and back to the USA.

"Those guys are such amateurs. They won't know what hit them. And they're even gonna train me to take their place after I whack 'em," Bruno was sure that his ship had just come in.

Pulling into their own driveway, Von Stein spoke for the first time since Bennette's house. "You are full of surprises, Carlos. Was that bomb for real?"

"No Señor Wolf. The real bomb is in the controller if he uses it, it will blow his hands off and make a large hole in his chest."

Von Stein was comforted to know he was in such competent hands. He felt more friendship for this complex man than he let on. In his mind, Carlos was a true oxymoron. An instinctive killer who lived by a code of fearless honor that few could understand.

CHAPTER 9: SERENITY IN THE E R

After an overnight rain shower, the air in New Mexico carried the fresh smells of the sagebrush and pinon trees. Juan Pedilla took another deep breath and put his shoulder hard against the tailgate. The old Ford Ranger pickup started to give way to the blacktop beneath it, slowly moving towards the graveled pull out. Juan was upset that his son had run the gas out of the pickup, but only because it was making him late for work. His son was a good man and also used the truck to get to work In the Pedilla family, everyone was working for a common goal, to buy they're own bean farm. Juan had worked for other people all his life and had been presented by his boss, with the chance to buy a hundred acres and the house his family shared. Mr. Shepherd was retiring and breaking up the ranch, selling much of it to his trusted employees and the balance to and Eastern mining company.

As the right front tire started to roll off the blacktop and sink into the gravel, Juan heard the sound of a vehicle approaching. "Bueno," he thought, "another farm hand is coming. That means help moving this Ford off the road, and maybe, they even have a can of gas with them."

What was coming was not help. In fact, it was a nightmare come true for Juan. Rodney Smith was blacked out at the wheel of his new Lincoln Continental. Rodney was a fifty-nine year old drunk with a stack of DUI tickets to prove it. The judge in Santa Fe had taken his license away over ten years ago, but that didn't stop Rodney. He drank like a fish and drove when ever he wanted to. Even six months in jail didn't stop him. The Sheriff had towed away three cars so far, but Rodney had plenty of money, so another car was only a phone call away. This fine morning, as the sun was rising, Rodney was returning from a three day drinking spree in Albuquerque. Blacked out from too much gin, his body was on auto-pilot careening through the foothills at seventy plus miles per hour on a forty-five mile per hour road. In his state of mind, he never saw the white Ford pickup. He did not feel the crash that projected him through the windshield and into the arms of a waiting tree. He hadn't heard the younger man scream just as the Lincoln met the Ranger, smashing through Juan's body like a paper cup on a railroad track.

Juan saw, heard and felt all those things, as if his mind was disconnected from his body. He felt the heat of the motor at his back. He heard the bones in his own body cracking and breaking sounding briefly like popcorn in a microwave. He saw the shower of glass as Rodney flew past him. He even recognized Rodney. Juan never lost his consciousness as the Lincoln bumped the Ranger over the hill and drug him thirty-seven feet before pinning him to the end of the guard rail section. He will always remember how happy he felt when the big V-8 of the car burped and died, then it was all pain. Immense, red hot all consuming pain. Then and only then, did he pass out. 'Amazing Grace' started playing in his head and then nothing.

Jackie was already six hours into a twenty-four hour shift with the trauma team when the call for the Lifeguard helicopter came in. It had been a slow night thus far at the University Hospital Trauma Center, the only level one trauma center in a four hundred mile radius of Albuquerque, and, although slow nights happen, they are rare. As Jackie was an advanced RN, with cross training as a flight nurse, she was put on stand-bye status when the regularly scheduled flight nurse came down with the flu. She had been trying on a crisp new blue flight suit when the call came in, so all she had to do was pull on the white flight helmet and run for the chopper.

Brian Paterson, the pilot had the rotor blades spinning slowly as Jackie reached the landing-pad. Brian Green, the copilot was removing the tie-downs. Everybody referred to this flight team as the 'Double B Team'. Jackie just called them 'Pat and Green'. This morning was Jackie's seventh trip out with the Double B Team, and only her twelfth trip as a flight nurse on the helicopter. The procedure is much the same as an ambulance, except the ride is much smoother and the trips generally shorter. Jackie loved to fly, the experience seemed to heighten her senses.

"Where to?" she asked Paterson after plugging her helmet into the communications port.

"Sounds like a bad wreck a little east of Espanola," The pilot returned.

"How many involved?"

The pilot flipped some switches before answering. "Two that I know of, maybe more. I'll tune us all into the local EMS boys after we're air borne."

Jackie looked around the interior of the Eurocopter A-Star. Although she knew the Heli-Dyne Systems EMS interior was several years old, it looked brand knew to her. Even after daily use, the flight crew kept the A-Star in perfect condition inside and out. She made a quick inventory of the trauma supplies while the two Brians did the pre-flight check, returning to her seat just as the machine started to move. As she buckled her seat belt the craft rose softly, then tilted forward, stuttering slightly in the prop wash, then moving off and up as the rotors grabbed 'clean air'. Although Jackie's stomach seamed to do a back-flip every-time they took off, the ride was superb. The city quickly fell away and Jackie felt an excitement build in her. Once on the ground she would assume the responsibility for the triage at the scene. Protocol dictates that the flight nurse has final say on who rides in the helicopter and who goes by ground ambulance. It is at times an awesome responsibility. A decision that could very well mean that one person lives while another dies. Jackie took such matters with the proper amount of seriousness and thrived on the pressure, and although her sponsor advised against it, she really felt that her ability to stay calm under stressful situations was her strongest suit. The red and white Lifeguard helicopter turned north, with the morning sun sitting on top of the Sandia Mountains on Jackie's right. She asked for help from her higher power in making the correct decisions this morning.

Back in Albuquerque, other emergencies were happening fast. An ambulance was careening through the morning rush hour traffic with a cardiac case. The attendant feverishly trying to save the elderly mans' life. He had apparently collapsed on his stationary bicycle in the suburb of Rio Rancho.

Even more seriously, another ambulance team was arriving at University Hospital with two gunshot cases. Victims of a gang feud over drug sales turf, both young men where in critical condition. The ambulance had announced a 'hot arrival' to the trauma team by radio, meaning that time was critical in saving the lives of these teenagers. Neither the paramedics or the trauma team knew that a car load of gang-bangers were following the ambulance to the ER, intent on settling the territory dispute for good.

Eight people from the ER met the two gunshot victims and whisked them inside just as the heart attack case showed up in another ambulance. The paramedics unloaded their patient by themselves and called for help as they went through the door. Extra help had been called in and four residents were arriving to help the trauma team. Two of the resident student doctors took charge of the cardiac case, moving quickly to try and stabilize his condition. The ER had come alive with activity.

Outside of Espanola the Santa Fe county deputies had marked out a 100' by 100' landing zone about sixty yards from the crash sight. Brian Paterson expertly maneuvered the rotors between the cliff and a high power line.

"You're senior member, Jackie. That makes you the boss today," Brian Green said as they touched down.

Jackie already knew that as a trauma trained flight nurse, her status gave her charge over Brian Green who was both a pilot and a paramedic.

"My pleasure, Green. You take the guy from the tree, I'll take the smashed guy." The men on scene had reported a few basic details while the rotary craft was in flight. The local ambulance team and deputies had carefully removed Rodney from the tree with the use of a backboard and had laid Juan prone next to the guard rail that had stopped him from going over the embankment.

"We didn't want to move him too much," A deputy said as Jackie knelt next to the victim. "His name is Juan. I know his whole family."

Just then, Juan came to for a moment. "An angel," he said, then was gone again. Jackie, took a quick breath to stabilize her own emotions, and was thankful that he was passed out. His body was an obvious mess. The less pain he felt, the better. She quickly checked the ABC. Juan's airway was okay but his breathing short and shallow. Probably broken ribs. Not too much blood was evident for this much trauma, however, internal bleeding was a grave concern with this kind of accident. A quick listen with a stethoscope revealed that Juan's heart was regular, but elevated.

"Let's get him on a back board. He'll make it if we can get him to the ER in time."

After moving Juan to the board, Jackie cut away his clothes to better assess the damage to his legs. Both legs were broken in several places. It appeared that his left hip was shattered. The Cadillac emblem was embedded low on his back and bleeding in an oozing manner. Jackie was now sure of internal injuries. She instructed a local paramedic to start an IV and carefully place his neck in a brace. Then she stepped over to the other victim.

"What'ya got, Green?"

"Multiple 'lats'. Broken leg. None of that's too serious, but I'm afraid he might have a broken back."

After a quick check, Jackie turned to the sheriffs' deputies. "Show me what happened here. Run it down precisely, don't leave anything out. And show me that tree."

The men complied more efficiently than she had hoped for. All the information was processed by her well trained mind, helping her to make the only decision she felt comfortable with.

Jackie called Paterson on the helmet radio. "Brian, I saw how tight that was coming in. I hate to do this to you, but we really have to take them both. Can you get out of here with that much weight?"

"Affirmative, we are at five minutes, twenty seconds." The Double B team had a reputation for lift off in less than seven minutes from touch down.

"Okay, people, listen up," she stopped all of the action around her with her commanding voice. "We are taking both. This one is fragile with a probable broken back. Start him for the chopper now. Carry him, don't roll him, slowly. Six men. Go now."

She returned to Juan. "We can roll this man. Let's load him before the other one gets there. I can do the most good for him in the aircraft."

As soon as a man was loaded into each side of the A-Star, Brian Green strapped the victims down for the ride and waited for Jackie to insert an IV needle into Rodney and a second IV into Juan, then signaled Paterson. The aircraft lifted slowly and smoothly up past the power lines, shifted sideways about two hundred feet and started to climb, gaining speed as it went. Green was always amazed by Paterson's performance as a pilot. It was as if the huge, heavy machine had moved on a fixed wire. So smooth that it was impossible to tell the craft was moving at over a hundred miles per hour in just a few seconds. He keyed his mic.

"What do you need me to do?"

"Get a cardiac monitor on the back case, cut his cloths off and re-check everything you can on him. Then call his condition in to the trauma unit. I want to keep my full attention on this one, he's got more broken parts than I can count. I'll call him in, in a few minutes."

When she turned back to Juan, his eyes were open again. For a brief second, she could feel his pain.

"Juan can you hear me? Do you know what happened? Do you know where you are?" His eyes seemed to brighten, but he said nothing. "You had an accident. I'm a nurse and you are on the way to the hospital in a helicopter. Do you understand?" She could see he was trying to form a word. She removed her flight helmet and bent over, putting her ear close to his mouth.

"Amazing Grace," was what she heard him say, however, she had no idea how she could hear a whisper inside the noisy A-Star. A tear leaped from her eye as the first line of the song burst forth in her mind, blanking out all other sensations except one. She could feel his hand squeezing her own in a desperate attempt at communication. As his hand slackened, her awareness returned.

"Stay with me Juan. You are a macho hombre and your family needs you. You can do this. We can do this together!" His eyes closed just as she released a heavy dose of morphine into his system. Jackie flipped the switch so that her headset microphone was on the trauma center frequency, and called in Juan's status.

In Albuquerque, the trauma team leader, Nancy Bickworth, took Jackie's call. "We'll be ready," she said, and stepped over where Dr. Stalin, the trauma surgeon and the head of the trauma department was frantically directing the doctors and nurses administering to the two gun shot cases. Lots of decisions were being made by him in an unending stream of commands.

"Nancy, take the one on the left and head him for the OR."

Just as her team started to move into the hall with the patient, a strange metallic sound rang out. It wasn't a sound anyone had heard in this ER before. It took a few seconds for the first person, an x-ray tech with a military background, to identify the sound as that of an AK47 being chambered. He yelled 'gun', but it was too late to warn anyone. Shots thundered across the trauma center.

Three young Asian men, armed with an AK assault rifle and two handguns, had opened fire on the two gunshot victims with no concern for the nineteen healthcare workers attending them. Twelve people took bullets, including a fatal shot to the chest of Nancy Bickworth.

The two police officers who had come in with the gang victims came sprinting from the lounge, where they had been filling out reports. They both drew and fired at the gangbangers as they rounded the corner. The two men with handguns dropped dead. As the man with the rifle turned, a security guard hit him from behind with a high flying tackle. The Ak47 skidded across the floor to the feet of the cops. The entire event took less than ninety seconds. Three people had died. Eleven had been wounded. All had been horrified.

Dr. Stanlin rushed to Nancy, hoping to find life. There was none. Her heart had taken two 'cop-killer' rounds at close range. It looked as if he could put his fist into the hole.

"Okay, it's over," he yelled. "Check each other out, see how much damage was done to us. We're all professionals. Help each other." His mind was racing, almost out of control, his two years in a MASH unit in Viet Nam came rushing back to him. The fear, the carnage, the horror he had seen and the miracles he and his staff had to accomplish. His stomach turned into a hard knot and his mind became crystal clear. Triage and delegation is what Viet Nam had taught him about unexpected emergencies. Triage was difficult at the moment, but one thing he knew, a whole lot of people needed to go to the OR for surgery. He and Dr. Smith, the one other surgeon on duty had to get to work in the operating room quickly to try and save as many lives as possible. With Nancy Bickworth gone, someone had to stay in charge. Jackie was the only other person with enough experience to direct traffic so that these student nurses and interns could do their jobs efficiently, and right now, efficiency counted.

"Where's Jackie?" He said not looking up, but expecting someone to answer. "Did she get hit? I need Jackie, now!"

"Jackie's on the Lifeguard flight, ETA-four minutes," an intern said.

"Okay, listen up. Dr. Smith and I are going to OR. Someone call communications and have them call in at least two more surgeons. I don't care if they're on the golf coarse. Someone go to the pad and meet Jackie. Tell her she is in charge down here until a staff doctor or senior nurse can take over. The rest of you quit whining, patch yourselves up and save these other people. If you are hurt too bad to be effective, lay down and stay down. Don't get in the way."

Dr. Stanlin started pushing one of the original gunshot cases towards the elevator, Dr. Smith had the other one loaded and was holding the door. Stanlin felt the panic settle in his throat and made it go away with a few deep breaths. This was no time for him to loose control. He looked down and noticed for the first time that his patient had a new hole in his shoulder with blood leaking onto the floor. The severity of the situation grabbed his heart like an iron claw.

"Give us a little help here, Lord, we need a break and we need Jackie."

As the helicopter crossed the city of Albuquerque, Jackie's thoughts had settled down. She wanted to make sure that she was giving proper care to both patients, knowing that the guy with the broken back, who reeked of alcohol, was probably at fault for this horrible accident. It was not her place to be judgmental and her training both in AA and as a nurse taught her to accept things as they were and just deal with them. It does no one any good to get too caught up in fault finding and accusations. However, it was hard not to be bitter about alcohol reaching out and ruining the lives of these two men. There really wasn't much they could do for Rodney while in flight, unless he woke up. She just had to make sure that her motives and priorities were in line, and they were. She made ready to deplane while Brian Green called in their arrival.

Two nurses assistants met them at the heli-pad. One helped Green to unload Rodney and the other was helping Jackie with Juan.

"Glad you're back a few minutes early, we need you in the trauma unit. Dr. Stanlin has put you in charge until he comes out of OR."

Jackie didn't bother to close the side door on the A-Star. "Why, where's Nancy?"

"We had an incident a few minutes ago. Some gangsters came into the unit and shot up the place."

"Are you telling me that Nancy got shot? Oh my God!"

"Yes, Jackie, she's gone. I mean dead," the young nursing student started to cry.

The news hit Jackie like a bullet, her knees went weak and she started to falter, then, she remembered that the dying man in front of her was more important than her feelings. She steeled herself.

"I'm sorry, Nancy was my friend, too, but if I'm in charge, my first order is to pull yourself together."

"I'm sorry, oh Jackie, it was horrible," they were speeding the gurney down a hallway.

"We have to save these two people before we can allow our feelings to come out," Jackie's tone was kind but stern.

"Okay, but there's more. Several of the staff were shot, too."

"Oh no. Jackie said as they turned the corner into the unit. They scene was like something out of a gory movie. Lots of blood. People sobbing and yelling. It didn't look like to much was getting accomplished. She gulped loudly, stepped away from the gurney and clapped her hands three time as loud as she could.

"Attention everyone! Hey everybody, shut up and listen." The ruckus slowly died. "I'm in charge here. If you're hurt get out of the way and be quiet. The rest of you need to give me information quickly and calmly. I don't care what happened, we need an assessment of capabilities and then we need to triage, then we have to act accordingly. I'll ask, someone answer me, please. And please, no talking."

All eyes were on Jackie as if she had split the sea. "How many residents here?"

Six hands were raised. "Anyone specializing in backs?"

"I do." Answered a resident named Burt.

"Okay, take Brian Greens patient."

Burt and Green moved Rodney into a cubical.

"How many RNs? One twenty-three year old stuck her hand in the air. "Okay, you're on Burt's team."

"Does anybody have a count on the gun shot cases."

"I count three dead, eleven wounded, six of them look bad, and then there's the two civilians they took to the operating rooms," replied the single x-ray tech that was unharmed.

Jackie turned to a resident named Karen Stills. "Dr. Stills triage the bad ones, and Dr. Clinton take the others, Ben you take my patient. The rest of you divide up and help the residents. Is that a coronary you two have over there?"

"Affirmative," said one of the young doctors busy over the man from Rio Rancho. Jackie didn't know the two doctors helping him, but it didn't matter. They had continued to work on the old man. Even during the shooting, Jackie learned later.

"Lets get busy people, help is on the way but we don't want to loose our 'golden hour'."

As she shed her blue flight suit, revealing her green scrubs underneath, Jackie updated Dr. Ben Carter on Juan's condition. Then she called for x-rays and a CT scan. Next she set up an assistant to run communications. Along with the general calls for assistance from the various departments, she ordered an orthopedic surgeon for Juan. Grabbing a clipboard with a yellow pad, she then went from bed to bed gathering information moving assistants and CNAs around, ordering lab services, and organizing the technical support as needed. A few stern words about the bodies being in the way of saving lives convinced the two policemen to move the dead and worry about protecting the crime scene later. Twenty-five minutes later, help started arriving. Juan and Rodney disappeared into the hospital for labs and surgery, as did the others, one by one.

One hour and fifty-two minutes after the shooting, the trauma center assumed a normal pace. Jackie was relieved for a break by a tall blond staff doctor that she hadn't met before. University was a huge hospital, it was almost impossible to know everyone. She poured herself a cup of coffee and walked to the office of Katherine Deerfoot, the personal director and her AA sponsor.

Jackie sat the cup down and started shaking uncontrollably. Katherine reached in a drawer and grabbed a chocolate bar.

"Here, eat this. It will calm your nerves," Kathy threw the candy across the desk to her. "Tough day, huh kid?"

"It was horrible. So much carnage at once. Just when I thought I was used to the worst, someone changed the rules on me. It's not fair."

"Someone said you were in charge of the trauma center. That's quite an undertaking for an alkie."

"Hey, it wasn't my choice, just my duty. It was starting to fall apart by the time I arrived. I hope I didn't screw anything up. I'm not sure I could take it if my decisions cost some poor guy his life."

"Yeah, well, this is a hospital with a level one trauma center that gets all the worst cases for New Mexico and eastern Arizona. People die in a place like this every day. You can only do your best. But I worry more about you, every time that I see you ending up as a wreck over what goes on out there. The ego part of an alcoholic may thrive on the adrenaline rush, but the bruised heart of a person in recovery takes everything too personally. That could lead to depression and the next drink. You know that, don't you?"

"Well, what else can I do?. I am a nurse, and a good one at that. I think."

Jackie's nerves were calming a bit. It always amazed her that a chocolate bar was to an alcoholic what a half a Valium was to most people. Kathy's words of reason were beginning to sink in after this recent experience. A well trained nurse is welcomed in any department.

"You know, you are usually right. I guess that's why I love having you as my sponsor. The Double-B guys have been after me to be a permanent Lifeguard nurse. I love the flying and seeing the scene that created the mess that we have to transport."

"Yeah but, it's still a high stress job. How about pediatrics or the delivery room? Something where you can see good come from what you do," Katherine leaned back in her swivel chair, put her moccasin feet on the desk and sipped her own coffee. She always wore a modern version of Indian footwear to remind her of where she came from. "As your friend, I'm telling you, girl. You are flirting with danger. Don't forget this program is life or death for you."

"Okay, okay. I'll give it some serious thought. It's just that I feel that I need all this stuff, right now. It makes me feel like there's some kind of point to this life of mine that God has so graciously restored."

"If you don't mind me saying so, I think you have been trying to fill some sort of emptiness in you ever since that guy Larry disappeared. I thought you said you were going to turn that over to your higher power and get on with your life?"

"I've tried but..." The phone on Katherine's desk rang, interrupting her thoughts. She wanted to tell Katherine about her trip to see Larry, but this wasn't the time, and besides, Larry had said not to tell anyone.

"You better get to a meeting when you get off or I'll come drag you there by your hair. It's an old Indian trick, very effective," Katherine said as she picked up the phone on the third ring. Jackie waved and left the office. Glad for the friendship, but not in the mood for the lecture.

The rest of the day was uneventful. In the trauma center emergencies came and went. Several people thanked Jackie for her efforts in sorting out the mess after the shootings, but for the most part it was business as usual and she went on about her job. Around five in the afternoon she was sent on a meal break It felt like a long time since that chocolate bar she had for breakfast. The excitement of the day had used up all of Jackie's energy reserves. She suddenly felt as if her stomach was going to eat itself if it wasn't fed right now, so she took a generous helping of some sort of casserole and a large milk. Her friend Suzie G. was waving frantically for her to join her table. Walking across the cafeteria, she smiled at the fact that Suzie had three young male interns entranced with her charms.

"You boys haven't been drooling on the table, have you? I expect a sanitary place to eat, you know."

They all flushed, but a tall red head from Texas answered with a drawl. "Why no mam, we all just believe in paying tribute to a work of art." It was Suzie's turn to blush.

"Y'all have been very flattering, but I need to talk to Jackie, so would y'all excuse us. Pretty please," with a few bats of Suzie's false eyelashes she added the punctuation. The young men said their goodbye and disappeared through the exit door.

"So, tell me all about the shooting. I heard that you were in charge of everything," Suzie didn't waste any time when there was gossip to dissect.

"Oh, I don't know. I wasn't there for the big event," Jackie was tired of talking about what happened. This long after the fact, she was beginning to get resentful about it. She was tired, hungry and angry that her friend Nancy had been killed.

With a sigh she continued, "I didn't show up until seven or eight minutes after the fact."

The sarcastic tone of Jackie's comment shook Suzie's manners into line.

"I'm sorry, I didn't mean to be insensitive. The nurse that got killed, was she a friend of yours?"

"She was my mentor in the trauma unit for the last four years. It makes me so sick that those asinine druggie creeps would do such horrible thing to innocent people. I always thought the hospital was some sort of sacred ground. People who go to the trauma center have the right to expect sanctuary," Jackie was so angry that she was shouting without realizing it. She had the sudden urge to throw her tray on the floor and stomp around the room ranting. She held herself in check.

Suzie sat wide eyed for a second or two. "Wow, I didn't even know you could raise your voice. Maybe you should be talking to your sponsor instead of me."

"I already did," Jackie said realizing that others in the room were staring at them as if they were having an argument. "My turn to apologize. Guess I'm a little strung out. People have been acting like I'm some sort of a hero all day.

They just don't get it. Those guys killed one of us and did major damage to the unit. The doctors and staff saved all those lives. All I did was my job, just tried to put a little oil on the squeaky machine. Dr. Stanlin was the hero, he did seven surgeries in four hours. And Dr. Smith, and all those interns. Did you know that two interns saved a heart attack victim while all this was happening in front of them, and they never skipped a beat?"

All of a sudden, Jackie was overcome by it all. Tears flooded her face as she leaned into her hands. Suzie scooted her chair over and put her arm around her friend.

"It's okay. We all understand, it's just that people don't want to face the bad things that happen. They would rather talk about your heroism than Nancy's death."

Wiping the tears away, Jackie took a few deep breaths. "Thanks for putting up with me. I guess I needed someone to unload on."

"That's what friends are for, and as a friend, I think you would feel better if you ate your mystery casserole now."

"Okay," she took a bite and swallowed. "I feel tired and drained, now. My batteries must need charging."

The twenty-four hour shift was finally over at midnight. As she was putting on a light jacket, Dr. Stanlin asked her to stop by his office before she left. A couple minutes later she knocked on the frame of his open door.

"Oh, there you are. Please come in and sit down, Jackie." She complied. "I wanted to talk to you about this morning."

"Thank you doctor. Did I screw something up? It was such a mess, I just tried to follow my training."

"No, no, you were great. From what I hear, you probably saved several lives today." Dr. Stanlin was a kind sort of a man in his early fifties. "Are you all-right? Loosing a friend isn't an easy thing. We all loved Nancy. She will be missed dearly around here."

"It's hard, that's for sure. I just don't understand what's happening out there in the world. Never, in my worst nightmares, would I have dreamt this could happen here at University hospital."

"I try not to analyze it too much, just fix the ones in front of me and pray that they make a speedy recovery," he shifted in his chair and put down the pencil he had been absent-mindedly playing with. "This may seem too soon for you, but work goes on in a place like this. I would like you to consider taking Nancy's place as head of the trauma team on my shift," as he said this, he looked her straight in the eyes, searching for the answer that he wanted.

For Jackie, this was almost a last straw on top of a difficult haystack of a day. She had no answer, but of course, that wouldn't do. This was her boss, asking for her help. Her mouth was dry, her muscles ached and her head hurt. She had a cold feeling in her heart where the memory of a lost friend was fresh.

"Thank you for the offer doctor. I'm really tired, do you need an answer right now?"

"This is the end of our work cycle. Your answer can wait a day or two, but I'd like to know as soon as you make up your mind. You probably know most of the particulars of the job. There would be a big pay raise and the usual perks as a supervisor. It's a regular schedule of fifty-six hours, time and a half over forty. More over time optional. You would be in direct charge of the nurses and techs on your shift, coordinate the operation of the trauma facilities and do crisis management when called for, as you did this morning. Do you have any questions?"

Jackie was so overwhelmed that she thought she would cry again. "No questions that I can think of. I just can't make a decision like that on the run. It's a great opportunity for me and you must think I'm qualified, but, I'm not sure I can handle it. Let me do some soul searching after I'm rested. Is that okay for now?"

"Sure, I understand. We've all been through a lot today, but you know this business is twenty-four-seven. The emergencies still happen and the people who depend on the trauma services still need our best efforts. You are a big part of that, and yes, I think you are the best nurse we have in the unit now. We can pull someone from another department, if we have to. But you chose to work in this hectic environment, so you are the logical choice."

"Okay. I just need to rest."

"How would you feel about next week, even if your answer is no to the long term commitment? It would help me to know we were covered until things could be settled." "That would be fine, but I'll still need time on the big picture."

"Go home. Get some sleep and call me in a day or two. I want you to know how much we all appreciate you today. Thanks, from all of us."

Jackie sat on the edge of her bed, tears spilling over her eye lashes. She was too tired to sleep and too emotional to make any decisions. She needed rest and an AA meeting. Doctor Stanlin's offer was too big of a decision to make without talking to her sponsor and doing some major prayer and meditation work. For now, maybe a hot bath would help.

Lighting a candle for the dead is a custom in many societies, so she had a candlelight bath with soft music in Nancy's honor. Somehow she knew that Nancy would have liked that. Back when she was a drunk, Jackie didn't have to feel the pain of a lost friend or a death in the family. Now, such feelings were strong enough to leave a huge hole in her soul. It would have been nice if she could have called Larry, for some comfort, but it was impossible. She mourned for Nancy and all the lives harmed by the drug dealers and their ninety seconds of revenge.

Things didn't seem to be going well emotionally for her lately. First, just when she thought she found a man to be interested in, he disappeared Was it really possible to have a broken heart over someone you don't even know? The aching in her chest told her it was. Then Larry reappeared, sending her on a different kind of roller-coaster ride. Ever since her father had died earlier in the year, she felt alone in the world. Her Dad was the last surviving member of her immediate family. And now this stupid act of violence that would never be forgotten. How was she supposed to feel about it. It was an awful thing to have to carry around. How could she just step in and take Nancy's place. Nancy was the best nurse she had ever known. The pressure to keep it together and make all those important decisions would be like wearing an ambulance on your back.

Coupled with the grief, it was all just too much too think about. It pained her head to try and think. She was so tired that her face hurt and so tense that her back felt broken. Jackie turned her living room stereo onto a smooth jazz radio station and set the volume low. She eased back into her living room recliner with a comforter and stared at the candle she had carried back from the bath.

The mind can play some strange tricks sometimes. Her ears heard the pounding on the front door, but her mind just assimilated the sound into the dream that was in progress. It was a nightmare of sorts, but fun on it's own level. The dream was one of the drinking dreams that so many alcoholics suffer for years after their last drink. The dream took place in a posh disco, where, she was having a wonderful time. The music was loud and the drums had a steady beat that matched the pounding on the door. The Jackie in the dream had a great big frosty frozen mug of beer. It looked so cool and refreshing after all the dancing and fun she had been having. Just as she was about to take her first drink of the night, Larry came sliding across the dance floor, wearing a white three piece John Travolta suit, snatched the beer just as it was about to touch her lips. He threw the mug at the huge mirror ball and it exploded with a million refraction's of light and color. It became so bright that it hurt her eyes and there was a loud bang. Then several more bangs. The bangs became a pounding. Suddenly she sat upright in the chair and became fully aware of her surroundings. The incessant knocking had finally awakened her. She stumbled to the door, still under the intoxicating influence of the dream.

"It's about time, I've been knocking for almost ten minutes," Katherine's beaming face was framed by large beaded earrings with the thunderbird design. "I told you I would drag your butt to a meeting. I was just about to get the apartment manager to make sure you were okay. You better get dressed before the 'Great Spirit' gets angry with you."

"Well, good morning to you too. You know you aren't always so easy to take in the mornings. Please no Indian philosophy before coffee."

"It's not morning, white girl, It's five thirty. PM. Get your cloths on or will be late for the six o'clock meeting."

Jackie went to the bedroom and pulled on a pair of wranglers under her housecoat, feeling the effects of the dream starting to fade. She didn't want it to go.

"Wow, I've been asleep about twelve hours," she shed the robe, pulled on a T-shirt, tight jeans and slipped into a pair of sandals. Then she quickly ran a brush through her dark hair and washed her face.

"Okay, I'm ready."

Katherine shook her head. "How do you do that white girl?"

"Do what"

"You've only been awake for seven minutes and you look stunning."

"Well, if I had that natural Native American look, it would have taken a lot longer. Do you think your ancestors wore lipstick, make-up and jewelry on a daily basis?"

"Okay, you win. Come out to the reservation with me sometime and I'll make you an honorary Indian."

While driving to the meeting they discussed Jackie's new job offer. After hearing a logical view from Kathy, it just became crystal clear to Jackie that it was way too dangerous to her sobriety to add that much stress to her life.

"I guess that does it," she said as they pulled up in front of the High Plateau Alano club. "I'll call Dr. Stanlin this evening and tell him no, but I might investigate a little more about the flight nurse job. I really do like to fly."

"Take one step at a time, sweetie," Katherine turned off the motor. "We better get in there, I signed you up to chair the meeting tonight." The dashboard clock read 5:56. They rushed in to take there places at the table.

CHAPTER 10: CHIHUAHUA

It was the smell that captured Larry the most. That familiar smell. That exciting yet dangerous odor that rang alarm bells in his mind, as it was pulling him into the dark experience of the club. He and Cisco had been in dozens of bars and cantinas during the past few weeks. They had visited classy joints and dives from the tourist hotels around the plazas to the back alleys of Ciudad Juarez . All of them had triggered different types of memories for Larry, but this one had it all. The smell of booze and the noisy way drinking people conducted them selves. The odor of warm human bodies having a good time mixed with the faint smell of the poor ventilation from the rest rooms. And perfume, be it cheap or expensive, off set by cigarette smoke-all these things made this bar exciting. The lights were low and a hot salsa/disco band had a large dance floor packed. Every kind of clientele was here. He guessed the place probably held five or six hundred people. Another emotion that a big bar like this brought to the surface was the fear of the unknown. Anything could happen in a room packed full unpredictable drunks. If you were a stranger in a place like this, you had no way of knowing who the players were and which face was a mask of trouble. La Casa Verde was a huge happening place and it's ambiance was overwhelming to Larry. Before they could get to a table, Cisco noticed Larry was affected.

"Hey, Señor Sully, are you okay. You look a little pale."

"Sure, just a little tired, I guess. I didn't expect this big of a crowd."

Larry took a bag of M&M candy from his pocket and shoved a handful of the chocolate bits into his mouth. A waiter took their drink orders. Larry ordered a Coke in a can, Cisco a bottle of Carte Blanca beer.

"Hell of a place to try and do business. Don't tell me, one of those guys from the bull fight owns this place, right?"

Cisco paid for the drinks, which seemed to show up really fast for a busy bar like this. "You got it Señor Sully. I've heard that El Gordo owns it. Bringing us here to do business shows trust. That is good."

"I suppose that's true, but we are on their turf, again," Larry tried to not sound annoyed, but he would rather have meetings in a more controllable environment.

"Everywhere in Ciudad Juarez is on their turf. Relax, my friend, we'd be dead by now if they didn't like us."

Up stairs, behind a mirrored plate glass window, El Gordo-the Russian and Don Alonso sat in over-stuffed high wing back chairs and obseerved the crowd below. Both had cigars and large snifters of brandy. El Gordo, the Russian, leaned closer to the glass for a better look as he spoke.

"I see our American friend and his man are here. They look anxious to do business. I assume the trial transaction went well?"

Don Alonso sipped his drink thoughtfully. "If there was any discrepancy in their story or their behavior, they would be dead by now. I had my friends in the Mexican Mafia check them out. Señor Sullivan is what he said, a made man in the Las Vegas Mafia. I think he is trying to gain favor with the bosses by making a big deal for them. He just did a piece in jail for the good of the organization. I think maybe this is his way of showing respect and that there is no hard feelings."

"And the muchacho he travels with?"

"We double checked him, but we have known of him for years. He is Francisco Angle Garza Fuerte. He poses as a guide, but really he is one of the many "fixers" we have here on the border. He gets things done for people. Arranges a meeting one day, sets up a small drug buy the next day, and takes a rich gringo wife shopping on a third day. He makes a percentage on anything he does, and pays Groupa Diablo for protection. He is just an independent street hustler running after the gringo dollar all day."

"Bueno, my friend, let's bring in this representative of El Cigarro and see what he is like."

Don Alonso complied, although he had to suck in his resentment. He was an important man and did not like the way El Gordo gave orders when he easily could have phrased it as a request. The vast amount of cash that the Russian was willing to invest in Groupa Diablo had bought a certain amount of respect, but only as a minor partner. El Gordo would never have the power to command Don Alonso to do anything. Don Alonso nodded to his bodyguard and Bruno was ushered into the room.

Bruno was agitated, having been made to wait for over an hour, but knew how to act when a boss held court.

"Don Alonso, Mr. Bennette sends his greetings and prayers to you. Your reputation on the border shows much strength. I'm sorry that I don't speak your language, please forgive the rudeness of my English. My name is Bruno and I can speak for Don Bennette on any matter."

The Mexican felt better already. A man of his power needed to be respected. It was his way and his fathers way before him.

"Muy bien, tell me if you know the man in the cowboy hat and vest sitting next to the yellow pole."

Bruno stepped up to the glass and scrutinized the cowboy.

"I don't know this guy, should I?"

"No, but you will soon. He is a gringo Mafia from Las Vegas. His name is Tom Sullivan. He wishes to buy more cash than we can provide. That is why you are here."

"Yes, Mr. Bennette has a large supply of the cash we sent to you last month. How much does he want and what is your interest?"

"We believe he wants millions, over a period of time. We could broker the deal, but we think it is better for you to make your own deal with Señor Sullivan and pay us a finders fee and for transportation to the north."

"Thank you, Don Alonso. You show much faith in us, being that our operation in Mexico is new. What figures can I report to Don Bennette?"

"We will take five percent of the net amount for a finders fee and three percent will insure safe passage to El Paso."

"Don Bennette will want to negotiate, of course, but that seems like a fair place to start," Bruno's pulse was rising as he tried to figure his personal profit.

"No! Tell Señor Bennette there will be no considerations. Meet our price or we will just bury the gringo in the desert, and none of your money will go through Ciudad Juarez! Ever!"

Bruno was visibly surprised by the forceful nature of the Mexican warlord. El Gordo spoke for the first time.

"I'm sure Don Alonso means to have a long working relationship with El Cigarro, but this is Mexico, Bruno, you must learn the Mexican way of doing business. It is not much different than the way your bosses operate in New York and Chicago. Simply tell Mr. Bennette that he is a guest in this country and he is not in control. War in the high desert is swift and certain. There is much to be gained by agreeing to our offer."

"I will tell Don Bennette immediately."

"Muy bueno. We will sent the cowboy to Chihuahua next week. All the cash he buys will be delivered to us along with our percentage in clean money. Then we will transport it across the border for you. Comprende?"

Bruno nodded in respect and exited the room.

A few days later, Trevor sat in a quiet cantina during the siesta time of day. The warm sleepy sunshine gave him plenty of elbow room to review the notes he kept in a worn leather notebook that resembled a mans wallet. He had lost track of his subject, Larry. It was the first time since the beginning of the assignment that he hadn't known of Larry's exact location. He could only assume that Larry and Cisco had gone to Ciudad Chihuahua, to further their investigation. By following, eavesdropping and asking questions he was able to know almost as much as Larry. And Trevor knew that it was inevitable that they go to Chihuahua. The question was, how was he to go there without blowing either his or Larry's cover?

Trevor had been a 'border rat' for nine years. That's what the suits called undercover federal officers that worked deep cover along the more than two thousand miles of US-Mexican border. Formally a Marine, a police officer in Del Rio, Texas, and a US Customs agent, he now worked for all the Federal agencies. Just like Larry, his paychecks came from a blind consulting firm and his records were held 'sealed' in a vault in Washington DC. The big difference was that Trevor had a territory that he worked in continuously and had built an ironclad deep cover story. He really did judge minor rodeo competitions and he worked hard at being the conspicuous aging cowboy that this part of Texas was famous for. By being around all the time and so obvious, he became part of the scenery to the locals on both sides of the river. He knew hundreds of Mexicans by their first names, spoke pretty good Spanish, and was a respected story teller. Most people thought he was involved in some sort of illegal business, but nobody knew for sure what it was. In the bars daily, the locals never gave a second thought to why he never drank beer or booze. He always said the he had 'just had one' or had 'reached his daily limit'. What ever, he knew people were far more interested in themselves than anything else. Often enough, he purchased a round of drinks for his friends and nobody gave a second thought to his beverage being coffee or cola.

This current assignment, gave Trevor a lot of respect for Larry. Being in AA himself, he had an inside awareness of the difficulties the agent must be facing. He was told this guy was a top operative and that was almost an understatement. In a few short weeks, Larry had penetrated the bad cash ring clear to the top without taking any unnecessary risks, appearing both competent as an agent and comfortable with his new identity.

If Trevor waltzed into Ciudad Chihuahua as usual, Larry was sure to know he was following him. Trevor knew he could trust a well seasoned undercover agent like Larry, but it would not be good for Larry to have too many things to think about. Undercover work was about concentration, and the situation in Chihuahua was sure to be an extremely dangerous playing field. Still he was Larry's real caseworker and this was Trevor's operation from the start. He was also Larry's backup if anything went wrong-and they often did on this kind of assignment.

He decided to catch a ride with another undercover operative who flew planes for the drug traffickers, and then use one of his alter-ego disguises while he was there. A false nose so big that no-one dare look at his face, add a slightly worn priests robe, put a stoop in his lanky frame, and it was time for 'Father Minion' to visit the churches of Chihuahua.

Cisco was sitting in the pickup cab when Larry came down to the parking lot for their agreed upon six o'clock rendezvous. It continually amazed him that Cisco could change his identity so effortlessly. Today he looked the part of a slick Mexican 'narcotraficantes'. A brightly colored silk shirt, gray slacks, patent leather boots, several gold chains and a white shoulder holster with flashy pearl handled gold plated forty-five automatic. On the seat beside him was a M-16 combat rifle, canteen, and a large thermos of coffee.

"Hola Señor Sully," Cisco was using his thick accent with an intimidating sarcastic smile that would make you immediately not trust him. "I picked the lock, hope don't mind too much, Señor. If you do I could always kill you and your mother and have my way with your cat and your sister," Cisco laughed.

"Jesus, what are you supposed to be, a disco serial killer?"

"Don't get your knickers in a bunch, old boy," He switched to a British accent, then American. "In Ciudad Juarez it's best to be low profile but on the open hi-way the drug traffickers rule."

"Do you think we will need all that protection.?"

"Mostly just for show, did you bring your gun.?"

"It's under the seat, wrapped in a towel, you know if I get caught with it in Mexico, it's straight to prison," Larry had never mentioned the gun in his boot.

"For the trip, get it out and wear it openly. Our cover for the ride to Ciudad Chihuahua is that I am a trafficker and you are my 'pistolero'. Don't worry, the local cops are all asleep. I replaced your license plates with plates from the state of Sinaloa. That's where most of the traffickers come from, so we are just business men on a buying trip."

Trusting anybody while undercover was a hard thing, however Cisco had earned that trust the past few weeks, so Larry did as he said. Three hundred seventy kilometers of open desert lay between them and Ciudad Chihuahua.

They stopped for lunch at a roadside stand on the outskirts of El Sueco. Cisco made sure that the locals noticed his flashy new persona, it was good to create a memory The scenery was turning mountainous. Back on the road, the traffic was sparse, they would occasionally see American motor homes and RVs, traveling in a convoy for protection, and a few over used local cars, long past their prime and down to the primer on the paint job, inadequate mufflers spewing blue-black smoke.

A few miles south of town, an Army jeep passed them going the opposite direction. The jeep turned around and started to follow them at a distance as if they were waiting for something.

Cisco adjusted the mirror on his side of the truck. "They are going to stop us, just waiting until we get to a good place, probably a side road so they can take us off the hi-way, out of view."

"Please don't tell me this will be a shoot out."

"No, no. I know how to do this. These guys aren't for real. The two in the back have on Mexican army uniforms, the driver looks like a Mexican Federal Judicial Police officer. The other guy has on officer clothes with no insignia. Probably DFS, Department of Federal Security. In the real world these men would never be together. They are big rivals, but out here you can be the type of policeman you want for about twenty thousand dollars."

"It sounds dangerous to me."

"No, I got it covered. It's about respect and money. Let's pick our spot, pull over at that viewpoint up ahead. Don't say anything. If I get out of the truck, you get out and hold the M-16, but don't threaten anybody with it. Just keep your sunglasses on and look tough."

The men in the jeep took their time, stopping well back from the big four by four. One of the men in the back seat casually pointed his weapon at the truck. The front seat passenger cleaned his chrome sunglasses before walking up to Cisco's side of the truck. He was wearing a military army officers dress shirt, new wrangler blue jeans, boots, a three point officers hat and a nine millimeter pistol was stuck in his belt. He was tall enough to look down into the large pickup, maybe six feet four or five. The man flashed a DFS badge and credentials at Cisco, too quick to read, but that wasn't necessary.

"Hola Comandante," Cisco sounded respectful.

The man leaned in and made an obvious inventory of the weapons that were in plain sight.

"Expecting trouble?" The officer's English was good.

Cisco started into a nervous oratory, speaking Spanish so rapidly that Larry had too listen hard to keep up with the conversation. The man seemed bored with it all. Finally Cisco ask him to take a walk and talk about a problem. Maybe the Comandante could help. He exited the vehicle and walked the Comandante up the road about thirty meters. Larry climbed out of the cab and with the M-16 held in crossed arms and moved about twenty feet away from the silver pickup to improve his field of fire. Both soldiers in the back of the jeep got out. One stretched, the other lit a cigarette.

Larry tried to keep Cisco and the soldiers in view at the same time. It was hard to do and he was getting more nervous all the time. He set his jaw trying to look like a tough guy. About the time he realized that he couldn't remember how to operate the combat gun, he saw Cisco pull an enormous roll of cash out of his pocket, peel off about half of it and hand it to the Comandante. The tall man said something and Cisco handed him a few more bills and pocketed the bank roll.

Cisco motioned to Larry and they quickly entered the pickup and drove away. The jeep went the other direction.

"So you had to pay off the cops, huh?"

"It's the way things get done here, besides, they weren't real government officials. The only question is 'how important they think they are', so I know how much to pay. No problema Señor Sully."

"What about the money?"

"Don't worry about it, I have a rich uncle, you know, and he is interested in our safety."

Carlos was fully dressed in the basement room of the mansion that he used as a 'Dojo'. He was practicing a drop-roll-pull gun and shoot exercise. First with left hand, then with his right hand. The German entered the room in swim drunks and robe, having just finished his morning swim.

"Good morning, that looks dangerous."

"Only for the other guys, Señor Wolf."

"Listen, that Italian slob, wants us to go to dinner tomorrow. He is meeting with a new client and he wants me there. I don't like it, but he is ready to pay us off and collect the other half of the plates. This is a dangerous thing to do with strangers around. How ever, we need to go. Be ready for anything, my friend."

"Yes, Señor Wolf, I am always ready. Are you willing to carry a gun, Señor?"

"You know that I don't care for weapons."

"Yes, we have had this conversation before, at least try on a bullet-proof vest. I don't want to lose my friend after all this time. Porfavor, Señor Wolf, it is my job to protect you. Is it not?"

"All right, do you have something in blue?"

Pedro felt his age as he walked home from the Hacienda de Flores in the evening. His feet, back, and weathered hands all hurt about the same. Lately, he had been experiencing small pains in his chest. He didn't think that was a good sign. Dedication, stubbornness and now hope compelled him to go to work for the Italians every morning, and, everyday he walked home with the sunset, feeling like his life was slipping away. His biggest wish was to stay alive long enough to keep his promise to Don Roberto. The Italian devils needed to pay for their sins upon the Flores family and Pedro intended to be there.

Turning the corner into the alley where his apartment was, the gleam of a big silver four by four overwhelmed the old man. What now? Had God finally sent an angel of mercy or was death sitting at his table. The light was on in his room and he could hear voices. He didn't stop to think about it, what ever happened was up to God. He pushed to door open and entered.

"Uncle Pedro! How good it is to see you. Come sit at your table, this is the man I want you to meet. This is Tom Sullivan, he is the man I was telling you about."

"Pleased to meet you Don Pedro, please call me Sully. Cisco has told me many brave things about you."

"Thank you for your respectful greeting, but I don't feel like a 'Don', just plain old Pedro. The invisible gardener."

"From what I hear, you deserve a Saint-hood. Come sit with us and eat. Your nephew just had this nice diner sent over from the cantina so that we could eat and talk in private."

"Well, if you are our angel, then there is hope, and if there is hope, then I guess I might feel like eating again," Pedro sat and began to grin. Food was passed around and as Cisco and Larry explained the plans they had, the grin on Pedro's face got bigger and bigger until it seemed his face would crack. Now he knew at least some of his prayers would be answered.

The old man slept sound, restful sleep for the first time in weeks. His dreams took him back to the old days when the hacienda was the show place of Ciudad Chihuahua. Happy faces of four generations of the Flores family danced passed him in the finery of the great room. All of the important people who had visited the hacienda in the last fifty years waltzed by in turn. The women dressed in formal gowns with bare shoulders and the men in ties and long coats with tails. A group of his favorite children sat at the baby grand piano, playing for the dancers. He always loved the children, having none of his own. And behind the children stood his own beloved Esperanza wearing a blue gown much nicer than he had ever given her. She appeared at about age forty, tall, proud and beautiful. He took her hand and began to dance. The room fell away only to be replaced by millions of stars.

At the Ciudad Chihuahua airport, Trevor, dressed in his 'Father Minion' disguise, phoned for the cab of another old friend who was actually a CIA deep cover operative. The cab driver updated Trevor's knowledge of the local criminal elements on the way into the city. Trevor borrowed an old Ford surveillance car from the man and checked into the Hotel Plaza, an older cheap hotel that listed TV and air conditioning. As a priest, he didn't need to create a huge cover identity. Not many people questioned the activities of the clergy in this part of Mexico and Trevor always believed that 'KISS', (keep it simple stupid), was the best way to stay invisible. Armed with his Pentax camera and bag of telephoto lenses, he could be a priest on holiday and appear to be taking snapshots of buildings or birds while using a telephoto lens for a good look around.

Trevor was acutely aware of the need to be very cautious for Larry's sake. The CIA man told him where to find the Flores hacienda, so he drove passed it and took a few innocent pictures. He had a view of the front of the main house and did not count Larry's pickup among the parked automobiles.

A casual drive past the hotels didn't turn up the truck either. Trevor knew that it was an unusual car for this part of the world and would turn up soon-he hoped. It was necessary that he get on Larry's trail as soon as humanly possible. He had a bad feeling that his job as backup might make a life or death difference. About sunset he took a window seat in a side-street cantina and ordered diner. In his opinion, the out of the way local type restaurants were always better. It didn't matter which country he was in as he had acquired a taste for real Mexican dishes. As the sun shifted in the late evening sky, he caught a glimpse of silver with his peripheral vision. Leaning back so he could see between two ancient buildings, the silver took the form of a big four by four pickup. He finished taking a bite of his tamale and wiped his face. But he couldn't wipe away the smile. He knew he was good at this job, but sometimes it sure seemed that some power greater than himself was extremely helpful.

After dinning with Pedro, Larry and Cisco checked into the Hotel Soberano Chihuahua, a five star beauty that sported all the amenities that north Americans are used to. Larry used Tom Sullivan's VISA card for check in, renting two adjoining rooms. Then they went into the bar and ordered drinks, rum and Coke for Cisco and cranberry juice for Larry, paying with Sullivan's MasterCard. Larry wanted to be sure and leave as much of a paper trail to identify Tom Sullivan as possible. It had been a long day since leaving Ciudad Juarez, so they turned in about eleven o'clock.

The next morning they went for breakfast in the hotel coffee shop. Larry was wearing a western style light sport coat and cowboy hat. Cisco was decked out in another successful narco-trafficker outfit, as he called it with a tight red v-necked T-shirt gold chains and a dark blue silk shirt unbuttoned. Larry could see how well muscled his thin Latino body was, it reminded him of Bruce Lee. He wondered when Cisco found time to work out. The gold and pearl handle of Cisco's forty-five caliber was visible under the blue shirt.

"Don't you think someone might see that thing stuck in your belt? Isn't that dangerous for us. I always heard the state police threw away the key if you were caught with a firearm."

"Maybe for you, gringo," Cisco said as he pulled the gun and purposefully checked the clip, slamming it back into place with a loud snap. A lady tourist with blue hair gave him a disgusted stare. He pointed the flashy cannon at her and pretended to fire. She and her husband hurried out of the room.

Larry was instantly horrified. It took most of his reserve to keep from yelling at the kid and grabbing the gun.

"Hey, I don't think that's a smart move. Put it away, now, please."

"Trust me Sully. These are strange times. A tourist with a popgun would get arrested, but everyone is afraid of the narcos. Look around. Is anyone calling the police. Do you see the manager rushing to our table?"

The room was normal, as if everyone was pretending it didn't happen. The help went about their business, the customers studied their food. In a few moments conversations were back to normal. The incident with the golden gun was erased from history.

"Okay, you win your point, but I still don't think that was smart."

"Don't sweat it. It helps our credibility. Three or four good incidents, and everyone will know who we are."

"Well, we not here to become famous, or I guess I should say infamous. We just need to make this deal and get back to the border where we have a support net if we need it."

"Oh we don't need to worry too much about that. Fast Eddie has a good network all over northern Mexico, and Pedro isn't my only relative in this town."

"Still, this is worrisome for me, being in a foreign country and all."

"Speaking of back-up." Cisco's tone turned serious. "You know that cowboy we kept bumping into. Well, I took the liberty of putting a couple of Fast Eddies guys on him. Looks like he might be some sort of a FED. He had a meeting with a red headed government type a few days ago. They followed the red head into the Federal building in El Paso. He went into the Treasury offices."

Larry was slow to respond, giving time for his brain to catch up to his emotions. This was not a time to loose control over this operation.

"You should have consulted me first. I never told you that I was working alone. Your men just wasted their time." He saw the pieces of the puzzle come together in his own mind like a movie that you weren't allowed to understand until the last scene. He had a basket full of issues to sort out about this, but not now, not here, and definitely not out loud.

"Hey, I was just trying to do my part. I didn't think you knew. You must be better at this than I thought."

Larry wondered. He had been concerned about Trevor, but every time he would start thinking about, he couldn't get past the AA angle. It was like the AA part of his brain said he had to trust certain people even when his years of experience said otherwise. What Cisco said was a reminder that slapped him in the face with the cold wind of reality. He wasn't paying quite enough attention to business, and that, could be fatal.

Don Alonso said that they would be contacted at the hotel sometime in the morning. As they were finishing breakfast, three men appeared at the coffee shop door. A large Italian looking guy with a black leather coat was flanked by two men with Uzzies slung under their jackets. On the left, a red head that was so Irish looking you could almost see a shamrock in the freckles on his fore head. To the right a large Mexican with a clean shaved head and sunglasses. Larry steeled himself and dropped his arm across the edge of the table so that his hand was only an inch or two from his 9MM Glock in it's shoulder holster.

After surveying the room, the trio crossed the room towards Cisco and Larry. They stopped in front of the table, one gunman facing each direction. The drama seemed so staged that Larry almost laughed.

"Mr. Sullivan, my name is Bruno. You are to come for diner at the Bennette hacienda this evening. A car will come for you about six."

Larry turned in his chair and opened his hands in a gesture of friendship that also deliberately showed the gun in the holster.

"Can I offer you breakfast or coffee?" Larry didn't wait for an answer. "A car isn't necessary, we know the way. Be sure to set a place for two 'cause we'll both be there." Larry deliberately put on his sunglasses.

Bruno could see his own sardonic smile in the mirrored lenses.

"Right," Bruno made a mock gun with his fingers and fired it in the general direction of the table. "Be there, no second chances."

"Gotcha!" Larry smiled big. "Please extend my greetings to Mr. Bennette. I'm looking forward to our meeting. We may know some of the same people, you know."

Bruno grunted like a tough guy, turned and led the rough looking bunch from the dining room. Larry turned back to Cisco and tried to be serious but Cisco laughed out loud, making Larry grin.

"The Italian Mafia must think this is still the nineteen fifties or sixties. Can you believe those guys? The sunglasses were a nice touch. I think Bruno was genuinely hurt that he couldn't intimidate you."

"You liked that, did you? See, it isn't always necessary to pull a gun to be a tough guy. I've dealt with mob guys that would make Bruno pee in his designer boxers."

"Maybe that's why they sent you on this assignment."

"Could be. I don't know, but those old muscle heads are so predictable that it's like watching a movie for the third time."

Cisco stood up and smoothed his silk shirt.

"I think I'll nose around a some and see if I can find out anything we don't know. Do you want to come."

"No, I'd just slow you down and my Spanish isn't that good to keep up. I'll just hang out here and concentrate on the meeting."

"Okay, I'll be back before five. Adios."

Rosa let Pedro into the house, via the kitchen, during the afternoon. He went immediately downstairs to the servant's quarters and moved a huge plain armoire away from the wall in Rosa's room. It was old and very heavy taking all the strength the old man had. Behind it was a passage into a small vault, about five feet by six feet.

Pedro wiped the dust off of a turn of the century steamer trunk. The kind with a rounded top. Opening it up, he lifted out a large black sombrero revealing several family journals, some silver ingots, a few pieces of family heirloom jewelry in a small wooden box. At the bottom two forty-five caliber 1870 model colt pistols, complete with holsters of fine carved leather and silver, lay on top of a maroon Mexican gentleman's suit. The suit included a laced linen shirt, embroidered short jacket and tailored britches with silver conchos down both legs.

It was the outfit that Don Roberto wore on cattle drives when the cattle were driven into town for sale. He had also worn it when he played a bit part in a movie about Pancho Villa.

Pedro carefully lifted the guns and clothing, and laid it all out. From a corner he picked up an old bottle of tequila from a case lot. Popped the cork out and held the bottle up to the clothes as in a salute.

"Tonight, my old friend. Tonight I will keep my promise to you."

He took a long swig from the bottle. He was in no hurry, he had several hours yet.

Room service brought Larry a pot of coffee about two in the afternoon. He had skipped lunch, spending his time going over all the details of the case so far. Feeling that this was a secure room and not having any plans to go out, he filled a yellow legal pad with notes of everything he could remember. Starting with the objective of the operation, Al Bennette, then everything he knew and guessed he knew about Tom Sullivan. The character had to be played right at diner. East coast mob people were always testing and evaluating people, trying to trip them up-the consequences of which was death. He had to assume that by now Bennette or his men had talked to Chicago and Las Vegas about Sully. It was a big leap of faith, but he had no choice but to trust agent Smith to have given him the correct data.

Taking his time to make sure that all the parts of his cover story and what he was going to introduce into the situation matched, he rehearsed answers to potential questions, being careful to never speak louder than a whisper. He compared the process to a lawyer preparing a defendant to take the witness stand in a capitol murder case. Every nuance had to be right. Years of government undercover work had given him a built in memory bank full of details about crime figures and important cases. The same kind of details that the older mobsters in Las Vegas would have told Sullivan about the good old days. Bennette was sure to be filled with ego about being one of the characters in a few of those stories. Everyone, especially men who think they are powerful, love to talk about themselves to anyone who'll listen. It was Larry's security blanket, and he was well trained to play this game. His fear was that every champion on a game show gets beat sooner or later.

Having worked through this sequence by the time his coffee arrived, he turned his full attention to the problem that had been growing in the corner of his mind all day. Trevor. Friend or foe, cop or not, Trevor could be as useful as a handle on a suitcase or as dangerous as a bomb in a box. And what about this AA connection that Trevor had cultivated with him. Was it real? T sure knew his Big Book stuff. That part had to be for real. It seemed unimaginable that the government would assign two recovering alcoholics on the same case. But then again his own sobriety was still fairly knew. What if the law enforcement agencies were full of recovering people and he had just failed to notice. It wasn't a stretch to believe the 'Feds' had someone watching him. It had been expected and if so, he was glad if it was Trevor. The guy was likable and he felt he could probably be counted on if the crap went through the fan. Putting his feelings of resentment and possible betrayal aside, he decided to put it in Gods hands for the moment and take a shower followed by three aspirins and a nap.

Bruno always got the job done. That's how he got to be a 'made man' in the Chicago Mafia, and, that's how managed to stay alive. The bosses said that, 'to put Bruno on someone's case was like putting a Pit bull on their butt'. He would sink his teeth in and never let go. He wasn't a very intelligent man, but he had the ability to focus on one thing at a time. At the age of sixteen, he taught himself to read and write, something that the teachers hadn't accomplished. His uncle Vinny was in the mob and said if he couldn't read, he had no future except to carry a gun and be the first to die. The Mafia had moved into legitimate businesses and was using more college graduates and even computers. Bruno hadn't made college but he moved up the ladder because he understood respect, and never let them down.

This new venture with Al Bennette was something different for Bruno. He had never had a chance to act on his own, however, he felt that the Chicago bosses had let him down by sending him to Mexico with this raging drunken mad-man. In his mind, he deserved a measure of compensation. A Mafia Don could take Al Bennette's new money making scheme as an offense and kill the whole bunch of them, or, maybe the bosses would be understanding an just ask for their cut. With all his heart he felt he was doing the right thing and hoped the bosses would be reasonable when they found out. Of course, he could always skim his retirement money from Bennette, then turn Bennette into the Chicago Dons and end up an important man himself. With Bennette out of the way, Bruno would be able to run the Mafia in Chihuahua. Maybe even build a personal empire. Don Bruno. It had a nice sound to it. All in all, he would rather go home to Chicago. Mexico was just too uncivilized.

Bennette was going to have him kill the German. No big deal. He'd just have to take care of the body guard first. That Carlos was a slippery guy. Obviously a qualified professional. Bruno understood about having the offensive advantage versus the defensive reaction. Much better to just shoot the guy in the back than risk getting shot yourself. Murder isn't fair. His deep thoughts were interrupted.

"Is everything ready for tonight, son?"

"Yes boss, three extra men inside the house and our bank people will be standing by their computers to make the transactions."

"Get those lazy whores dressed for diner, and don't let them take too many drugs this time. They are suppose to add class to the table, not pass out in the food."

"Okay, we brought them new dresses from the city today."

"Are we going to do the German tonight, boss?"

"Sure. Sure, just wait until this Sullivan guy leaves. Did you say he looks like a Mexican? Wonder how he got a 'mick' name."

"He is supposed to be the child of an Italian Don's daughter with an Irish gangster for a father. One of those marriages to end a turf war. The say Don Giancanti attended the wedding before the couple was sent down to Vegas."

"Get me a drink, would ya, son."

Bruno crossed the room, scotch bottle in hand and poured.

"You're a good boy, Bruno."

Stuffing his anger, he managed to answer.

"Thank you, Don Bennette," Bruno nodded and left the room.

If there happened to be gun play and Bennette got killed in the process of killing the German and Carlos, well, that would just be too bad. Bruno knew he could arrange it, but such devious actions could easily backfire. Could he really trust his men? Could he be certain that Bennette didn't have someone in his corner, watching, waiting to see where Bruno's loyalties lie? What if Bennette only got wounded? He would be exposed and Bennette would have him killed one way or another. Too many things could go wrong. He had seen friends die for smaller schemes back in the windy city. It's best just to bide the time and see what happens. The only way to loose in this situation was to be too greedy. He decided to have a little fun with one of the Mexican women before the guests arrived. That would take his mind off of these greedy thoughts.

After driving to a secluded spot in the city, Trevor opened the trunk of the CIA car. He was pleased to find that it had been fitted with a false bottom containing a few 'spook' goodies. A quick inventory showed a twelve gauge sawed-off shotgun with a modified magazine that held sixteen shells, two forty-five caliber automatic Colts, a Mini-Mac nine millimeter machine pistol, a fancy H-K sniper rile, a Kevlar bullet proof vest, night vision binoculars and a parabolic microphone for listening at great distances or through windows. His friend had loaned him the right car, not only all the goodies in the trunk, but also a modified high performance engine and heavy suspension to make the mid-seventies boat corner like a cop car.

While Cisco and Larry were talking to Bruno at breakfast, Trevor was across the street listening through the parabolic, picking up every word. Afterward he followed Cisco for a while then doubled back and found Larry to be inactive. Feeling he had enough information about the meeting with Bennette, Trevor decided on a little rest himself. He had a feeling it was going to be a long night and he wondered if Larry really knew how dangerous the situation was. A certain fact was that Trevor was there to watch Larry's back, weather Larry knew it or not.

Returning to his modest hotel room, he slipped off his priests costume and opened his Big Book. He read pages eighty-four through eighty-eight, about the promises and asked for knowledge of God's will and protection from his own selfish will. He wanted this Bennette guy to go down hard, but not at the expense of Larry or Cisco. Trevor laid back on the bed and tried to visualize the different possibilities at tonight's meeting and how he could fit into what ever went down. Some how he would be there.

CHAPTER 11: DINNER GUESTS

Driving into the hacienda, Larry and Cisco made many of the same observations that Carlos and Von Stein had made on their first visit, counting manpower and weapons, noticing escape routes and line of fire zones. Larry didn't like this part of the job. He had been away from the tactical part of police work for much too long. Although most undercover work has an element of danger to it, most of it is up close and personal, with back up of an entire government agency or two just a quick phone call away. Sometimes, it's just a holler or a nod, and the cavalry will come charging in. But here, in a foreign country, with just himself and this cocky kid and nobody to call, the odds were starting to spook him. It was becoming harder to tell himself that he was just here for information while he was counting AK47's, and the tough guys who planned to use them. He had stayed alive this long by sticking to the Boy Scout motto, 'Be Prepared', and this was no time to get sloppy.

"Do you carry a back up?"

"You mean like the one in your boot?" Cisco was always a step ahead. "No Señor, not like that. My back up weapon is my mind and body working in unison."

"You trying to tell me that you're into Kung Fu or something? How good are you?"

"Only a black belt, in three different disciplines."

"Well, I hope I never have to see it." Larry again wondered how Cisco ever found the time for all the things he did. "How did you know about the hide away gun?"

"Just a guess, I've seen too many American movies. The good guys always have a second gun. It always saves their butt in the end of the film."

"Don't laugh, but I usually don't carry any kind of gun. It's my cover, this Tom Sullivan guy, that carries the two guns."

"Ah, I knew you'd admit that you weren't Sully, sooner or later." Cisco only stated what was obvious to him. Larry didn't flinch, he knew that the kid knew who he really was, it was just professional courtesy to keep up the façade between them.

They were met at the main house by Bruno with two Italian looking goons. Both had sport coats and turtle-neck shirts with shoulder holsters. The standard Mafioso enforcer costumes.

"We are glad you came gentlemen, may I put your guns in a safe place?"

"No thank you." Larry sidestepped Bruno and moved through the front door as Cisco opened it. The Mafia tough had no choice but to follow them through the door, loosing all power over the situation. Larry stood in the foyer, waiting for Bruno to catch up and post his men.

"Your boss is expecting us, is he not, Bruno?"

"Mr. Bennette and I are partners. He is having refreshments on the verandah. This way gentlemen."

"Oh, I see, Bruno. Your end of the partnership is to play messenger boy and butler." It was a crass thing to say, but Larry thought it would be in character for Tom Sullivan and keeping this big oaf off balance was good strategy. The real Sully had a reputation for a sharp tongue.

Stepping through the genuine French glass doors, complete with crystal door pulls, Larry was stunned by the spectacular view. Bennette stood with his back to the house, leaning on the stone railing that overlooked the flower garden and the city beyond.

"Our guests are here, Al," said Bruno, trying not to sound like a butler.

"Welcome to my little house on the hill, Mr. Sullivan." Bennette extended his hand. May I call you 'Sully'? And this must be Cisco, the boy wonder from Juarez."

"Yes, Mr. Bennette, meet my partner, Francisco Fuerte."

"Buenos noches, Cisco. You can both call me Al." Bennette seemed both uninhibited and relaxed. "Fix yourselves drinks and let's get aquatinted before our other guests arrive. I've heard that we both know some of the same people in Chicago."

"Cisco, would you do the honors, please?" The Mexican turned to the out-door entertainment bar and poured Larry a cola over ice and opened a beer for himself. Larry sat in a high backed white wicker chair. "Ya, I've been to Chicago and if you want to waste our time quizzing me about it, I'm sure my memory won't fail me, but if you hadn't checked us out, we wouldn't be here. Right?"

"Okay, okay, I believe who you are. No harm in talking about the good old days, is there?" Bennette noticed the lack of alcohol in Larry's drink, true to his information about Tom Sullivan.

"Well, Al, most of my good old days are memories of Las Vegas. It's my father who you would really want to talk to about Chicago. Can we talk freely here?"

"Oh sure, no problemo in my house."

"I don't mean to be disrespectful. We're here on business. The men on the border said you were the one to help me with my special needs."

"You are referring to large amounts of a certain kind of cash I presume?"

"That's right. Can you provide a sum as large as this?" Larry wrote '$250,000 per week' on a napkin and showed it to Bennette who handed it to Bruno.

"How many weeks do you want?" Bennette showed no emotion. Not a flinch.

"I can guarantee eight to start, then we will adjust to the usage factor."

"The amount is no problemo, but if we are doing that grand of business, I need to know more about it, what the motives are, who the players are, ect." Bennette poured himself another scotch.

Just as Bruno was about to join in, one of the goons appeared in the doorway and motioned to him. "Our other guests are here." They both disappeared into the house.

"You probably know that I just got out of jail. I did my time for the bosses like a good soldier. I don't want to start over again in the Las Vegas organization, so I thought I would take a gift back to them."

"You are a smart man, Sullivan. So what's the mystery?"

"Sitting in my cell, I realized that I'm in a unique position for a deal that is bound to happen sooner or later. My last task for the mob was as a liaison to the Native American casinos in ten western states. I showed them how to train the right people for management, invest their money, avoid tax problems and make sure that they were making enough money off of the gambling. The people I work for in Vegas thought it was better to make friends out of the new Indian gaming industry instead of enemies. We also provide personnel for security, supervision, dealer schools and technical support. Here's the angle. I personally know most of the top casino people in the Indian gaming industry. Tribal Councils, chiefs, casino operators and the like. No one else is privileged to all of those contacts and all that information across America. Not even an Indian."

"Okay, I follow that. It puts you in the sweet spot. So what?"

"I've made contact with a few of my Indian friends, and they are all eager to make an extra profit margin, and as you might guess, they aren't willing to share it with good old 'Uncle Sam'. After all these years, most of them still carry the grudges created by the treaty breakers of the old west. So I've arranged to sell them your money, which they pay out in small cash winnings, you know, five dollars to a thousand dollars, the real money that they take in, is treated with the normal amount of respect. Taxes paid, payroll, ect.. The bottom line is they can afford to pay out more winnings which means more business for them. The mob gets middleman money and I, being the only man alive who can do this deal all at once, get a boost up the food chain."

"Sounds like a plan to me, but can just a few casinos take that kind of cash without getting busted?"

"Most people don't know because the Native American casinos are pretty low profile, mostly, just advertised locally, but in the ten states that I dealt with directly, there are one hundred thirty-nine Indian casinos. Sooner or later some funny money will get back to a bank and the cops, but human nature is for people to hide their winnings and the casinos can claim they are being hit by the bad money as well. At the figure I gave you, it comes to less than two grand a casino per week, to start. Totally acceptable at even twice that figure. Distribution is simple 'cause we already have our people in place in all of the casinos. Also, much of the money is played back to the house, making it even safer to have large amounts of funny money on hand."

"You really have this worked out don't you? You should come down here and work for me."

"And eliminate the organization as a middleman. I'm not that brave, Al. You know what happens to those who break their vows to the Mafia. Now I've told you my story, what kind of assurance can I get from you. I'd like to be comfortable knowing that you can provide me the same quality merchandise, week after week, that I saw in Juarez."

"Well, Sully, here's your assurance now."

Von Stien was being ushered through the glass doors by Bruno with Carlos trailing behind, gun in hand as usual. The German was wearing a loose fitting white suit with a dark blue shirt with light blue tie. In his hand he carried an expensive leather attaché case. Carlos wore his custom made dark gray blazer with his usual working arrangement of hidden weapons. The outline of his bullet-proof vest was clearly visible between his well muscled body and the black T-shirt.

"Welcome, Mr. Wolf." Bennette acted the most confident host. "I'd like you to meet Tom Sullivan and his, ah, partner Francisco."

Larry stood up and extended a firm grip. "Howdy, do they call you El Lobo down here?"

The German started to roll his eyes, then noticed Larry's sincerity. "No, not to my face anyway. I won't let them." He shook Larry's hand and nodded to Cisco who was stationed a few feet away, leaning against the bar with his hand on the butt of his pistol. Cisco's eyes were on Carlos's weapon. "Don't let Carlos spook you Francisco, it's just his rather formal bodyguard training."

"A man can't be too careful, Mr. Wolf. Mexico is a beautiful but wild place. Have you been here long?" Larry tried to take an easy tone with the new arrival. Although he hadn't expected a third party in his negotiations, he had to be ready for anything.

Von Stien responded. "I've been here a while, but I've had a body guard most of my life. An old family tradition, I'm afraid." His aristocratic German accent was obvious.

Bells, whistles and sirens went off in Larry's head. He had heard of a European counterfeiter who called himself 'Wolf' from other cases he had worked on. He stuffed his surprise at finding such a juicy catch here in Mexico. No one told him this assignment could involve such high levels of crime. The stakes just went way up, and the danger had just increased ten-fold. He glanced at Cisco to try to convey the seriousness of this event, but there was no need.

122

The kid had transformed himself into a smaller copy of Carlos in the time it took to step away from the bar and put on his sunglasses. He sighed audibly, pulled out a cloth as if to clean his sunglasses, but instead, he pulled his golden 45 caliber from it's holster, made a display of polishing it and assumed the stance Carlos always took. If it hadn't involved guns, someone would have laughed. As it was, the only one who acknowledged the humor was Carlos who smiled slightly, his eyes hidden behind his own shades. Each man recognizing the seriousness of the others profession. If size were the only matter, Carlos could chew Cisco up and spit him out, but with what Larry knew of Cisco, he thought such a contest would be more of an equal match.

"May I?" Von Stien motioned towards the bar.

"Certainly, help yourself." Bennette drained his own glass, thought briefly about resisting another drink, then joined the German at the bar.

"Mr. Wolf is the reason we are all here tonight," announced Bennette. "He is the creative genius, as they say, behind the works of art you wish to purchase, Sully."

Von Stien stopped his drink halfway to his mouth. He had never expected Bennette to cross such a line of confidentiality. Such a indiscretion was considered crude, even among thieves and down right dangerous.

"Now don't let Mr. Bennette mislead you, Mr. Sullivan, I'm just a small cog in the large wheel he turns." The German made a feeble attempt to move the subject off of the obvious.

"You can call me Sully, and if you are the artist who made the bills I saw, my hat is off to you."

"Don't be modest!" Bennette said, his tongue starting to sound a bit thick. "Yeah, he made'em. And they're damn fine, if you ask me. That's why I, or we, bought his operation. The best quality I've seen."

"True, Mr. Wolf?" Larry had to force himself to concentrate on the conversation at hand, instead of the bigger implications. The information could be dissected later. Right now his job was just to collect the information.

"Yes, I'm afraid so. Al and I made a deal some time back and I have been training his people to run the entire operation with Bruno as the overseer. The training is complete now and we are about to finalize the deal." It was more information than the German would have liked to tell, but Bennette had opened this can of worms and Von Stien just wanted to get it over with and get paid. He was becoming more uncomfortable by the minute.

"Well, Bruno, are you happy with the training?" Bennette sat down hard in a wicker chair that seemed to groan with his bulk.

"Yeah Boss, it's not so hard if you got the plates." Bruno poured himself a rum and coke, wishing he could sound more like a partner than a hired thug.

"If both of you guys are good to go, then I don't see why we can't complete Mr. Wolf's deal right now." Bennette knocked over his empty glass as he gestured. "Bruno go warm up the computer and dial up the satellite link"

The German's face flushed red, then paled again. He certainly did not like his business known to strangers, but completing all dealings with the Italian scum-bags was good news; if he and Carlos could stay alive. Von Stien addressed Larry and Cisco, hoping that they were not on Al Bennette's payroll.

"Why don't you gentlemen join us and see how easy it is too control vast sums of money if you have the right equipment."

Bennette labored out of his chair. "Okay, let's do it."

The Italian led the way, as Von Stien and Larry met eye to eye for a few seconds, both men deciding, 'friend or foe'. Both choosing the latter.

In the sitting room, with all the modern gadgets, the atmosphere was extremely tense. Larry and Cisco were not sure of what was going to happen and the German was a figure of ice-no emotion, no expression, all concentration. Every muscle Carlos had was tensed for action, which made Cisco more than a little nervous. Al Bennette was totally relaxed in his well oiled state, but Bruno was pacing about like a cat on the hood of a Mexican cha-cha wagon at high noon.

Larry sat back in a high backed green velvet chair and tried to look relaxed while Cisco positioned himself opposite of Carlos at the door. Von Stien sat on the sofa and opened his brief case on the marble coffee table. First he took out a brand new laptop computer and opened it, then he pulled out the plates, each one wrapped in purple velvet. Bennette had plopped into an overstuffed Lazy-boy rocker.

"Are you going to inspect the merchandise?" The German adjusted his glasses.

"I'll let Bruno handle it. That's why we been schooling him, ain't it?"

Bruno put in a jeweler's loop and held each plate under a light for inspection. Cisco noticed that Carlos took the safety off of his nine millimeter when Von Stien had opened his case, so he did likewise. It was the subtleties in dangerous times that could save your life or get you killed.

At the sight of the plates, Larry felt the excitement of the moment well up inside him until it almost overwhelmed him. These people and these plates were the reason he was here, and they had just given him everything he needed to make a case. The location of the plates and all the players. If he could just make a couple of phone calls, he could get Bennette extradited and send in the federales, with an American advisor or two, to be sure the plates were 'returned to the US as evidence'. It was the kind of day a cop lives for, if he can survive it. He could feel that something was just not quite right. It was in the air and most definitely in the tension of the moment. God, he wanted a drink.

"I believe we should use both our computers to make the transactions." Von Stien held out the cord for his laptop. Bruno took it and hooked it up, then brought Bennette's laptop across the room and sat it next to the Germans.

"Go to this web site and put in the access code XDQ?/4(7wkjs6waD." Von Stien handed Bruno a piece of paper with the web site address and the code.

"Where did you come up with a code like that?"

"It's a new sixteen symbol computer generated code. Very secure."

Both the German and the Italian had "ROYAL CAYMAN BANK" on their screens.

"This is the account number." Bruno was handed another paper. He entered the number and an un-named account page filled the screen.

"All-right, we are ready, boss."

Bennette waved his cigar to indicate the go ahead as if he did this everyday. Bruno typed in $2,500,000.00 in the deposit blank and entered the account it was to be drawn on and his secret PIN number. Von Stien watched on his own screen as the transaction took place and his deposit balance increased by two and a half million dollars. Bruno carried his laptop back to the desk and quickly typed 'save' and hit the enter key, telling his computer to capture Von Stein's information. Later he would call up the account, after the Germans' timely death, and transfer the money back into Bennette's account.

Von Stien had his own plan. He waited, cleaning his glasses as a diversion, until Bruno had signed off line, and had turned off his computer, then typed 'GO' into his own machine. A preset program transferred the money into three different Swiss bank accounts automatically. He did the shut down procedure on his laptop. German team one, Italian team zip.

"There you have it. The modern age of the rich and shameless. Thank you Al, it has been a pleasure doing business with you." Von Stien felt like throwing up after telling such a lie.

"Well, that was quick, is there some sort of ceremony that goes with it." Larry tried to be deliberately sarcastic.

"It's the modern age, Mr. Sullivan. Millions can be moved from bank to bank in a blink of an eye."

Larry thought that was an odd thing for a counterfeiter to say. Maybe this German guy had more plans besides making funny money. It would be an awful loss if Mr. Wolf got away before Larry could alert any type of law enforcement. If this was the same person he had heard of, a dozen countries, at least, would be happy to put the cuffs on him.

Bruno put the printing plates in a medium sized safe that was inside a low cupboard. Cisco noticed that he locked the cupboard, but not the safe. Almost too easy. Arrogant men usually became careless.

Al Bennette led the group out of the sitting room, crossing the 'great room', to the dinning room by the terrace. The formal table was set with the finest china, crystal and silver. Several women sat waiting at the table like so many punished children. Vickie and Tina, Carlos' cousins, were spaced around the table with the last two Flores women, Emanuella and Esmerelda. The men sat and Rosa started serving at once. Bruno had barely sat when Bennette barked a command.

"Bruno! Don't just sit there boy, drinks for everyone. We must make a toast to the completion of our deal."

As he prepared the round of drinks, Bruno was seething beneath his evil smile. So much he wanted to be 'the man'. So much he hated his loud mouthed, drunken boss. How ever, he managed to tow the line and do as he was told. His time would come, no doubt about it.

When all present had a fresh glass, Bennette stood up, unsteady on his feet, weaving a bit and leaning hard on the table. He bumped a half full water goblet which tipped back and forth a few times without turning over.

"A toast to good business, lots of money, and, ah, ah, even more money. May we all get what's coming to us."

As they were all raising their glasses, the hidden door in the corner of the 'great room' banged open. Into the light stepped a spectacle from an old movie. Beneath a big black sombrero, stood the vision of a wealthy Mexican land owner in maroon and silver, holding two dangerous looking Colt 45's.

"Viva La familia Flores!" He yelled.

CHAPTER 12: TRUTH, LIES AND CONSEQUENCES

Jackie was cleaning out the back of the helicopter. It had been a long hard day. An eighteen wheeler had lost it's breaks on Interstate 40, coming down the Sandia grade into Albuquerque. Before sliding to a stop on it's side, the huge truck had caused a wreck involving fifty-three vehicles. It was a huge mess of humanity and steel. The morning commuters were backed up for miles and thousands of people were late for work.

A wreck of these proportions brought to bear the full capabilities of the emergency services of Albuquerque. Nine ambulances and two helicopters transported the massive amount of serious injuries. The 'Double B' crew had made seven trips to the trauma center at University Hospital with a multitude of injured victims. The inside of the air ambulance looked like a military hospital unit after a big battle. Blood, bandages, empty cartons, and spent hypodermic wrappers were everywhere. While one of the two Brians went to work on the small mountain of paperwork, the other tended to the fueling and maintenance of the expensive flying machine. Although the company had three helicopters and usually only had one on the flight line at a time, all three had to be ready to go at all times. Who knows what the next big emergency could be or when mechanical failure would strike. This left Jackie with the responsibility of cleaning and restocking the interior. She was nearly finished when she heard a familiar voice.

"Hi Jackie, I need to talk to you. Have you got a couple minutes." It was Suzie G., the young nurse that Jackie sponsored. She was wearing faded blue jeans and an old T-shirt with no make up. Her usually perfectly placed blonde hair was messy and pulled back in rubber band. When Jackie looked into her eyes, tears welled up in eyes that were already red and bloodshot from crying. Not the 'blond bombshell' look that Suzie usually portrayed.

Jackie wanted to grab her and hug away what ever the pain was, but knowing that she might have to play the tough sponsor role, she handed her a pair of rubber gloves instead.

"Here put these on. We can talk, but this work has got to get done. You look like hell, kiddo. Help me get this rig put back together and I'll buy you some dinner or something. Are you hungry?"

"I don't feel much like eating." Tears started to run freely down Suzie's' face, but she pitched in and started to clean one of the gurneys. They were both quiet for a few moments. Jackie wanted to let Suzie collect herself before getting into whatever the problem was, but the girl just kept cleaning and crying silently.

"Well, I guess you better tell me. What ever it is, it'll feel better to get it out in the open. Don't you think?"

"I, I, ah, I feel so ashamed! I really thought my life was going better than this. I feel so humiliated." Suzie started to sob uncontrollably.

"Than what? What happened?" Jackie sat down on the door frame.

"Do you remember that cute red headed Texan you met in the cafeteria a while back?" She said gasping for air between sobs.

"Yes, what about him. Weren't you dating him?"

She got the sobbing under control, for a moment.

"Yeah, his name is Scott. Last weekend I went up to the mountains in northern New Mexico with him, for a get away. His parents have a condo up there at Angel Fire. It started out so romantic, he seemed to be the perfect companion. We went horse back riding right away. He was just so cute, and that cowboy charm never shut off. By the time we went to dinner, it was late, I was tired and he had me mesmerized. I didn't even notice when he ordered wine with dinner. It was so weird. Like I forgot who and what I was. We were talking and laughing and eating. I looked down and there was a half empty wine goblet in front of me. My very first thought was, 'who drank out of my glass'. Then I had the horrible realization that it was, in deed, my glass of wine and it had my shade of lipstick on it. My heart fell, I went all dizzy for a few seconds after realizing what I had done. Then, I guess, the disease took over and some part of me said 'oh well, to Hell with it, at least I'm out of town, where no-one knows me. And I shouldn't make this wonderful guy uncomfortable by making a scene'. So, I acted as if nothing was wrong and helped him drink that bottle and another bottle of burgundy back at the condo."

"The next day we rode horses again in the morning, then went to a barbecue with some of his Texan friends. I had already slipped, so I didn't think it would make a difference if I had a few beers. My mind told me that I could always sober up later, but right now I could handle it. By evening I was feeling no pain when the hard liqueur and cocaine came out."

Suzie started sobbing, out of control again. Jackie, who was now seated across from her on the other gurney, reached out and rubbed her shoulder. She was able to continue in a few minutes.

"The thing is, that I don't remember most of the night, just bits and pieces. I'm pretty sure that I made a fool of myself at the party. They say that I was driving his new sports car when we left. I don't remember. Oh God, I'm a hopeless damn drunk, a real alcoholic! I just hate myself. The sheriff said I did these horrible things, but I don't remember."

It took a few more minutes for a new round of sobbing to subside.

"Sheriff? Tell me what happened. Are you in trouble?"

"Yes, I think I'm going to jail for a long time. I'm only here now because Scott bailed me out. I don't know how I can face him. I don't remember the accident. The police say I smashed his car into a tree and then left him there unconscious with a broken arm and an open head-wound. And me a nurse! How

128

could I do that? I must have walked down the hill into town because they arrested me in the bar. All I know is that I woke up, hung-over, in the county jail. It was so awful and I'm so ashamed. What will I tell my parents, they don't deserve this?"

She was sobbing almost to the point of hysteria. Moving over next to her, Jackie put an arm around her and tried to quiet her. After a few minutes Jackie got up and quickly finished her job while Suzie sat quietly.

A few minutes later, at Jackie's place, they decided on a pot of coffee instead of dinner. They sat across the kitchen table, talking for hours.

"I know how hard this is for you, kiddo. Do you have any clue as to why you had no defense against that first drink? You know it only snuck up on you because you let it. Did you learn anything?"

"I don't know. Right now I'm so mad at myself and ashamed about Scott's car and his arm. He may never speak to me again. But I know for sure that I can't drink anymore. No matter what."

"Scott can take care of himself. Didn't he know you were in the program?"

"No, I didn't exactly tell him. I wanted to retain my anonymity. I told him that you were my friend from AA, though. He could have figured it out."

"You mean, you thought he wouldn't think you were fun if you were in AA. Suzie this is about life and death, it's not a popularity contest. Lies and omissions just a fuel to the fire."

"Okay, okay, what do you want from me! I'm human too, you know? What am I going to do now? My life is over!"

"Well, let's start with how you really feel, and why. Was it worth it to give up your sobriety for a weekend fling with a cute guy?"

"Is that what you think I did?"

"No, that's what you told me you did. I think you just haven't taken this program seriously yet." Jackie poured another round of coffee, hoping for a little more honesty out of her sponsee.

"You know, I say a lot of the right things at meetings, or I try to, but you're right, I guess I've been doing a lot of half measures. I mean, I know that I'm an alcoholic and that my life with alcohol in the drivers' seat was crap. It's just that I thought that if I felt better, then, I didn't really have to do all those things that you and the others talk about."

"Do you still think that?"

"I don't know. Maybe things will be different now, at least I can see that there is a lot of work for me to do. And I can sure see that the way I was doing the program wasn't enough to keep me sober. I just hope I don't have to do the steps from a jail cell."

The conversation went on through two pots of coffee, a candy dish of chocolate, a bag of potato chips and some stale ice cream, then Suzie dropped a bomb on Jackie without realizing it. She was talking about the barbecue.

"And the guy who brought the drugs to the party was saying that stuff had been hard to get for a few months because some undercover cop named Larry brought down the whole supply route and busted some guy named Bumper Blue. He said that the cop had got in so tight with the bad boys-running' and gunning', drinking and drugging-that he had to go to AA to sober up. Everybody laughed at that. Then he said that this Bumper guy had a contract out on the dude. It was a big joke to everybody, but I thought about that guy Larry from our noon meeting. The one you've talked about. Do you suppose that he was this cop, and maybe he got rubbed out or what ever they call it? You said that nobody has seen him in a while and this could explain it."

Jackie's heart jumped into her throat. She felt suddenly weak and very tired. She let Suzie ramble on for a few more minutes, but really didn't hear much of what she said. When the blonde finally came to a stopping point, they made plans to get together soon to start working the twelve steps all over. Then she shooed her out and sat on her bed crying for a while.

"This is stupid!" She thought. "I really don't know that Larry's in any danger, an I just saw him a couple of weeks ago."

She had said the same thing several times over the last few weeks, but it didn't change anything to say it. The same hungry feeling was in the pit of her stomach every time she thought of him. It must be love, and understanding love isn't easy. And now the thought that he may be in real danger or even killed, was so upsetting to her. Oddly, for an alcoholic, she had no desire to drink over this situation. A few years ago, a hang nail would have set her off. The misery of it, oh poor me. The tragedy of it, oh poor me. Why are they doing this to me, oh poor me. Oh poor me, pour me a drink. On second thought make it a double and leave the damn bottle. It was time to call her own sponsor, and so she did.

Katherine had invited Jackie to attend an AA meeting out on the Zuni Indian Reservation near Grants, New Mexico, about eighty miles west of Albuquerque. It was good to get out of the city for a while and meetings in strange places could be exciting. They made the trip out in Katherine's' Jeep with the top down and just listened to the wind, enjoying the desert. For the trip back they put up the top so that they could talk. After discussing the meeting for a while, Jackie turned the conversation to what was bothering her.

"I know you think I'm a lunatic for pursuing this stuff with Larry, and I know that you must be tired of hearing about it, but, you're the only one I can ask about this."

"Is this just the same old thing?" Katherine dimmed the lights for a trucker.

"No. I want to know if you know anything about him that you haven't told me."

"Like what? What's going on?"

"Well, I heard something that upset me and I thought you might be able to verify it."

"What now? I don't think that he is married, if that's what you're afraid of. I heard him talk about his divorce at a meeting once."

"No. It's worse than that. I know that he is really some kind of a cop. You know, one of those undercover types that they make movies about."

"So, what if the guy's a cop? Is that so bad? You see lots of cops in your job"

"That's not the scary stuff. What I heard was that he made a big case last year and took a lot of bad drugs off the street and so now, there's a contract out on his life. I know that the reason why no-one has seen him, is that he's working again. But maybe he's in grave danger or even dead."

Katherine passed a slow moving pickup with several Native American women in the back, wrapped in their traditional blankets. Faces lit by the stars and a full moon. She took her time to respond. Realizing how important this was to her friend and sponsee. Katherine had developed a strong friendship with Jackie, but she knew that people have gotten drunk over far less than the death or potential death of a lover. Or even potential lover, in this case.

"Wow, when you decide to find something to worry about, you don't mess around do you, white girl? You must be a little shook up. Don't believe in anything until you know the facts, and, don't forget that projection is just another form of expectation. I shouldn't have to tell you that expectations lead to resentments, and resentments lead to self-pity, and that can get you drunk fast."

"Don't you think I should try and warn him? I don't have anyway to contact him. Do you know who his boss or sponsor is?"

"I don't know anything about him being a cop or not, but Bob would know. He's his sponsor, you know? How do you know he's working, have you heard from him?"

"I didn't tell you, but we spent a couple of days together. He called and had me meet him in Ruidoso. That was a couple of weeks ago and said not to tell anyone, so I didn't, but now, I just had to tell someone and I trust you more than anyone else."

"Me, trustworthy? Okay I'm here for you kiddo."

"Yeah, well, I thought maybe you could talk to Bob for me."

"Why me. Why don't you just go up to Bob and say, 'Bob, I'm nuts over Larry and I want you to break his anonymity.'?"

"That's just it, Bob's a real old timer. Those kind of guys always do things right by the book. He probably thinks of me as a newcomer. You are more on his level, he might talk to you about it."

"Sorry, Jackie. You're on your own on this one. But Bob's not unapproachable, he works with beginner's a lot. Although you hardly qualify as a newby with four years of sobriety. He may not tell you just what you wish, but maybe he can set your mind at ease, at least a little."

Jackie gazed out at the night, wishing she was just a little bit wiser and a lot less fearful. The lights of the city glowed in the distance. She thought about the million or so people on the mesa who were going about their lives and not feeling the emptiness that she experienced. The 'not knowing', was one of the hardest things to live with. How many times had she turned this over to God, just to be right back to the same feelings?

"BOB'S O. K. USED CARS', read the sign. The car lot sat on the portion of Albuquerque's Center Street that had once been part of historical route 66. It had been a car lot for almost seventy years. Bobs' uncle, and namesake, had left him the car lot when he passed away during nineteen hundred and sixty-two. Bob had worked there since 1957. The office sat back off the street, an adobe building that had once been a gas station. The neon sign shaped like a Pegasus that used to adorn the front of the building was now a decoration behind Bobs' desk. Also behind the desk was Bob was looking out the back window with a cup of coffee in his hand. When the door opened, he swiveled in his big green leather chair to greet the intruder, his grin becoming more sincere as he recognized someone from the program.

"Howdy, young lady." He pushed back the large white cowboy hat that crowned his bald head.

"Hi Bob, do you remember me? From the noon group? My name is Jackie."

"Sure do. How could a lonely old cowboy like me forget a pretty little filly like yourself.?" Bob had never actually been on a horse, but he thought the cowboy routine gave him credibility as a car dealer. "What can I do for you 'Missy', need to up grade your ride. I give a special deal to folks in the program, all the money you got for a down payment and all the money you're ever gonna make for monthly payments. Throw in your first born and your inheritance, and we can put you in a nice luxury car with a full gas tank. Maybe a Pinto. What'd ya say to a deal like that"

Jackie was laughing by the time he finished the oratory. His practiced smile was some how disarming and she felt instantly at ease.

"Actually, Bob, I just came to talk to you about something. I know you probably have a lot of rules about what you are willing to talk about around AA, but I'm trying to find out something important about someone I think you sponsor."

"Would you like a cup of coffee? Have a seat, Jackie. In my opinion, serious talk means serious coffee. I'll make a fresh pot."

As Bob started to make the coffee, she took a look around the office. It was clean and efficient but old. The few cowboy memorabilia that hung on the walls-an old saddle, pair of chaps and several sets of spurs- added very little color as most old cowboy stuff tends to be brown and the walls were deep tan. The sixties style office furniture was in good shape and the desk was polished. Although there was no ash tray in sight, the room had that old cigarette smell that you would expect from this type of historical relic. She knew that Bob was a smoker, he must be keeping the ash tray in a desk drawer. It was becoming fashionable for non-smokers to over complain about smokers these days.

In a few minutes, Bob returned from the other room with a thermos-pitcher of coffee and an extra mug for Jackie.

"That's the fastest coffee maker in the west. Bought it at 'Wally-world' last month. Still can't believe it does its' thing so fast. Okay, we're ready. What can I help you with?"

"I asked my sponsor and she said to just come and ask you. I guess she assumed that you could judge for yourself how much you could tell me. I'm not trying to break someone's anonymity, just find some peace of mind."

"Well, she was probably right. There are a lot of paradoxes and contradictions in the program. Bill W. and Dr. Bob realized that being human, sometimes we just had to go with the situation and our gut feelings. They left us plenty of breathing room in this area. I assume this must be about some 'affairs of the heart', as they say."

"Yes, it's about that guy, Larry, that hasn't been around for a while."

Bob shifted his gaze out the back window where an apartment building was under construction. After a moment he turned back to her. His face, now serious, his eyes searching as if he could read her soul through her own. She blushed with fear. Fear that her worst assumptions were true.

"Larry is kind of a special case among us. He is struggling and doing his best. What exactly do you need to know?"

"Just before he seemed to disappear, we were becoming friends. I think there is going to be a lot more. Since he's been gone, I can't get him off my mind. Do you believe in divine events? Anyway, I heard some things that scared me, now I don't know what to think. But I, I, it sounds silly to say it this way, from a grown adult, but I think I love him."

He could see the tears in the corner of her eye and the truth in her face. It touched his heart, but he had to be very careful with Larry's secrets. As he understood from Larry, the right knowledge in the wrong hands could mean life or death in his line of work.

"Yes, I believe in divine intervention, divine relationships and that God, as I understand him, sometimes directs people lives to a happier place. Larry is a nice man. I believe he is a good man. I don't know what else I can tell you. What have you heard that has you so upset?"

"What I heard is that he is, or, actually, he told me he was some kind of a cop, and now I heard that there is a contract to kill him, you know like in the movies. My first fear was that he had slipped and was drunk somewhere, and too proud or ashamed to come back, but then he called me a couple of weeks ago and we spent some time together. Now I hear this other stuff and it's, it's......hard. I don't know what to do. Do you know how to contact him or who his boss is? He needs to be warned."

A single tear rolled off her cheek and splashed in her coffee. She tried hard to ignore it but Bob pulled a box of tissues from a drawer in the desk and handed it to her.

"Well, if I were to tell you that he wasn't a cop, I'd be lying. If I tell you the true nature of his life, I'd be breaking his trust and confidence. I can tell you that I talked to him a few days ago on the phone and I believe he was sober and in good health. He is,... let's just say he's out of town and hopes to be back soon. I do think, though, that most cops get threats once in a while, it's probably not much to worry about. Just business as usual for him. If he calls me, and sometimes he does, I'll tell him what you said. Does any of that help?"

She composed herself quickly. "Thank you, yes. I think I understand. Next time you talked to him, would you tell him that I want to see him as soon as he gets back into town?"

"Sure I will, and I'll keep this conversation quiet, if you will. The less people know about Larry, the better."

"Never happened. Thanks Bob!" As he stood, she jumped up and hugged him and was out the door before he could say anything more.

"Kids these days!" He said to himself. He reached across the desk and picked up the picture of his wife. Her picture always made him fell warm and fuzzy inside. He sat the photo down and dialed the phone.

"Captain Moffitt, please. Bob Smith calling."

CHAPTER 13: GUNFIGHT AT THE HACIENDA

Trevor leaned on the open trunk lid and considered the equipment inside, under the false bottom. He decided that the best tools to back up Larry and Cisco were the parabolic microphone and the Heckler & Koch MSG-90 sniper rifle with the ten-power scope. He had sniper training in the Marines and thirty years later he was still an excellent shot. He would just have to trust that the CIA or who ever owned the expensive gun had taken the time to sight it in properly. After slipping off the priest robe and stashing it in the trunk, he grabbed the hi-tech gear and headed out across the desert hillside to the hacienda on foot. The big man had worn desert fatigues under the robe, complete with combat boots and canteen belt.

Being tall was a huge advantage when you had to scale walls and climb trees. After a few minutes he was set up in a tree just behind the wall on the southwest corner of the estate. It was a great location. Right out of the sniper manual. He sat in the fork of the big cottonwood tree, almost in a classic shooters position, like those plastic army men he had as a boy. He could lean back against the main tree trunk and the gun rested in the fork of a branch. Just enough foliage to cover him, but not obscure his view. After tying the parabolic microphone to a branch, he put on the headphones and looked through the scope. At about a hundred yards, he could hear surprisingly well. In his field of fire inside the house was the dining room, part of what must be the great room, and the entry-way with the front door on the east wall. The group of men were just coming into the dining room with the usual small talk. Four women were already seated and an older lady servant was placing condiments on the table. The view through the row of large picture windows was great.

Trevor had just started identifying bad guys and counting potential targets when everything went to hell. The big Italian looking guy, who was playing bartender, had just sat at the north end of the table when the older man at the south end, probably Bennette, stood up to make a toast.

When the vision of a Mexican 'Grandee' appeared in the big room behind the dining room, Trevor almost laughed out loud. At first he thought it must be an entertainer, then he realized that the old man was waving six guns in the air instead of a guitar. Trevor sighted in on him and saw it was the old gentleman that Larry and Cisco had went to see. Not a target. At that instant the old man yelled and started to shoot up the place. The noise was so loud that Trevor had to rip the head phones off of his head before thinking about anything else. By the time he got back to the scope, everyone had started moving at once. Trevor looked for targets and could hear the screams of the women even without the parabolic. He saw Bennette take a bullet in the shoulder and go over backward.

The guy at the opposite end of the table pulled a gun, but Cisco whirled and kicked the gun from his hand. The big Mexican with his back to the window jerked bald a man from the table and down on the floor. Then he saw two targets come from a side room and run towards the table, sawed off shot guns at hip level. He took them both out in true sniper fashion, one bullet for one kill. The first shot hit one man in the forehead. At first it looked like a fly had landed between his eyes, and then in an instant pieces of his skull, gray matter and a blood came out of the back side of his head in a red cloud. Like something from a horror movie As he went down, Trevor controlled his own breathing, trying to slow down time while he worked the bolt. It's easy to make a first shot, but most second shots are missed because of over excitement. The other goon kept coming. Trevor shot him through the heart. It must have been a clean shot, not hitting anything but soft tissue. The 7-mm round went clear through him and the front door, leaving a beam of light streaming into the hallway.

Sweeping the scope back and forth across his line of fire, there were no other targets for him, save three women running towards the old man. Everyone else must be on the floor below window level. He put the head phones back on. There were sounds of women crying, at least two people were moaning and Al Bennette was cussing a blue steak, half the words in English and half in Italian. He waited for the eternity of about two minutes, then he heard a several more gunshots. A bit later, the front door opened and he saw Larry go through in a crouched position. A few seconds after that, Cisco burst out of a window on the south side of the building. The kid got to his feet quickly, crossed the garden and went over the wall, down the hill. Both of his guys were out. It was time to go. He let himself down from the tree and carrying the HK MSG-90, went looking for Cisco.

Bruno was still brooding about how much he hated Bennette. His hatred at this moment was as hard as steel and as deep as the ocean. When the old Mexican started shooting, it took him totally by surprise and he was slow to get a weapon in his hand, then, in an instant, it was gone. Everything was out of sync for him. Every move was too late. Then he felt the hot sting of a bullet graze his scalp and found himself on the floor. He couldn't understand what was happening. He couldn't catch up to the events around him. Women's dresses passed by his head. He grabbed and tore one of the dresses ending up with only a piece of cloth. Then he passed out. When he came to, a few seconds later, everyone was gone except Al Bennette, who was pulling himself up by a chair while using every cuss word on the planet.

"Oh, no you don't, you old son-of -a-bitch." Bruno reached the gun lying on the floor and fired into Bennette. The old man went back down, hard.

"Damn-it Bruno, why are you shooting at me?"

He fired another round and missed. "Your time is over, old man, it's my goddamn turn."

"But I treated you like a friggin' son, we can rule Chihuahua together."

Bennette rolled over to free his right hand. It had a snub-nose 38 in it. He tried to fire but Bruno beat him to it, shooting three more times and hitting Bennette's head with all three. Most of the face was gone.

"Stay down and die you damn crazy drunk!" Bruno started to get up on all fours, and then passed out again.

It was a few minutes later when he regained consciousness again. The battle was raging out side. He stood and wobbled to the front door.

"I've got to get out there and fight for what is finally mine. I'm the man in charge now." He said to a couple of corpses in the hallway. They didn't talk back. He went through the door.

Carlos was facing the great room and saw Pedro come through the same secret door that he had seen him use before. He recognized the gardener and by the time he realized that the man was a threat, the shooting had started.

"Get down boss!" He screamed as he reached out and grabbed Von Stein by the collar, pulling him over backward to the floor, chair and all.

As a body guard, his first instinct is to protect and survive. Gun battles are always won by the man who stays alive. Not the one who uses the most bullets. He fell on top of the German and kept him down flat until the initial shooting was finished. When he raised up, the two girls on the other side of the table, his cousins, were just slipping through the door into the kitchen. Larry and Cisco were gone. The other three women were going though the secret door like rabbits down a hole. Bruno was down and out. Bennette was struggling to get up and screaming in a tyrannical rage.

"What do you want to do, boss?"

"I'm in your hands, get me out of here. Right now!"

"Okay, lets go out on the verandah and circle around the north end of the house. Maybe we can get a jump on the men guarding our escape. Be careful, there is broken glass everywhere, señor."

He used his gun barrel to break away the remaining glass from a picture window and helped Von Stein through the opening. They crawled to the steps leading down into the formal garden and duck-walked down the stairs. Carlos noticed a lanky human form slip from a tree down behind the west wall. That made sense to him, as he was sure he heard rifle fire during the fracas. Someone had a sniper watching their back. He figured it was probably that guy who called himself 'Sully'. The Italians weren't that swift.

Gunfire was coming from the front of the hacienda. He surveyed the north side of the grounds. No immediate threats to himself or his charge, however, he had backed the Mercedes-Benz against the stable building on the north side of the parking area. Three shooters were using the German car for cover. As the two of them crept closer to the action, he could see that they had the American pinned down behind a huge planter, half way to what must be his silver pickup. It would be better if the American was dead, he knew too much, but Carlos could only do one thing at a time. The first priority was to get to the safety of the bullet proof car. He took out a second gun and made sure a round was chambered, Then he took out a flash-bang grenade, pulled the pin and handed it to Von Stein.

"Throw it on the other side of your car and follow me. RIGHT NOW!"

The German realized that the damn thing was live just in time to throw it as directed. It landed about twelve feet past the driver's door, exploding immediately. The closest bad guy fell from the concussion. The others naturally turned in that direction. Carlos was half way across the open ground before Von Stein knew he was moving. He was firing both guns as fast as they would chamber a round. When they reached the car, the score was German team plus one car and the Italian team minus three men.

The temporary slack in the gunfire aimed his way allowed the American to reach his truck. He sped away in a hail of bullets, spitting gravel all over the manicured lawn. All the shooters turned their attention to Carlos. As Von Stein unlocked the car door, Carlos stuck one M-9's in his belt and ejected the magazine of the other. He reached for a new clip, but was too late. Out of the corner of his eye he saw the falling motion of a man who had jumped from the stable roof.

Carlos turned quickly and tried to side step. The man landed on his left shoulder and as they both went down, Carlos made an awkward attempt to pistol-whip him. He managed to scrape the gun hammer across the attackers eye. The man screamed as his eye came out of the socket. A quick roll and Carlos was back on his feet. He kicked the man in the head and grabbed again for a clip. As he slammed it into the Beretta, a bad guy popped up in the stable window.

Carlos was in high action mode, the state of mind that he had trained for everyday for years. With his senses heightened, the action slowed down to a manageable rhythm for him. It is a state of being that only comes with hours of grueling martial arts training. He dropped and rolled, firing two shots at the man in the window, one of which found it's mark between the eyes. He loaded his other gun behind an empty oil barrel. The next ninety seconds were all done by rote for Carlos. Acquire target and shoot. Reload when necessary. Each bullet finding a vital spot and claiming a bad guy. He ran, jumped, dropped, rolled and spun. To Von Stein it was like watching a ballet. Seventeen shooters went down in the court yard, then Carlos threw a smoke grenade and sprinted back to the car.

Von Stein was in the front seat with the motor running. Carlos slide behind the wheel and headed for the gate slowly. He knew the armored car would be safe.

A shaky Bruno had spent most of this battle crouching behind a statue with his ears ringing. The Irishman who was in charge of the outside men had moved up to the planter that Larry had been behind.

"Blow the car!" Bruno screamed. "Didn't you put the bomb on the car? Blow the damn thing. They're getting away!"

The red head smiled as if he had just remembered and pulled the remote detonator switch that Carlos had built from his pocket. He was still smiling when he pushed the button and half of his body vaporized.

Bruno slumped down behind the statue of Don Sancho Flores on a rearing horse.

"Shit!" He said.

And there he sat, master of a hacienda full of dead people. His world was quiet but he still heard ringing. The hacienda was finally his, but his first thoughts were to get those guys. All of them. Sully, Cisco, Wolf and Carlos. The remaining hacienda guards were coming out of their hiding places and staring at their dead and wounded co-workers. He should have said 'let's go get the bastards' and mounted up in the jeeps for the chase, but this wasn't a movie. Everyone was stunned. No-one was quite ready for what had happened. Carlos had gone through his squad of shooters like they were school boys, playing with stick guns. The scene was a depressing view of broken tough guys. It would take a day to re-group. Then they would go after them. But for now, he just sat and stared until someone came and took him inside to lay down.

It was the squeak of the secret door under the stairs that alerted Larry. The sound was out of place, it just didn't belong with the surroundings and it put a warning chill down his spine. He turned to the right and looked past Cisco who was standing behind him. There stood Pedro in all his Mexican glory waving the two antique sidearm. The twin forty-fives looked huge and menacing. Just as Larry yelled 'NO!', the house filled with thunder. Pedro had started shooting.

Cisco was already moving. Larry saw him spin around like an expert kick-boxer and knock a gun from Bruno's hand. As the gun clanked to the hardwood floor, Larry was pulling Vickie and Tina down out of the line of fire.

"Crawl into the kitchen and try to escape out the back door. Go now!" He told them as he pulled the Glock and chambered a round. A crystal goblet exploded above his head. Larry peaked over the table in time to see a plate glass window shatter from Pedro's bullets, then Al Bennette took a round in the shoulder. The force of the impact knocked him backwards over his chair. The other two guests were down out of sight, but the servant and the other two women were running past Bruno towards Pedro and the staircase door.

Larry saw Cisco trying to make his way across the great room on his hands and knees. He assumed that the kid was trying to help Pedro, but Cisco had other plans. Just as Cisco reached the sitting room door way, two men came from the room on the opposite side of the front door. Larry had started across the south end of the great room and he dove for cover as the men raised their weapons. When he looked up again, the man closest to him was falling, blood and brain matter spilling from the back of his head. Then he saw the other one get hit in the chest. It looked like a clean shot through the heart. Watching him fall, Larry started to analyze what was happening, but it was too much information and the questions had no answers. A voice in his head said, "take action or die." And so he did.

The secret door was on the far side of the room about thirty feet away. The women had pushed Pedro back through the opening and the door was closing. As Larry crossed the room towards the door, he reached down to grab a shotgun from one of the recently deceased Mafioso's. Just then another bad guy burst in from the kitchen entrance to the great room. He fired and Larry felt the bullet pass the side of his chest. It must have gone through his jacket but missed his flesh. He should have worn his bullet-proof vest. Too late now. He dropped instinctively between the two bodies and another man opened up with what sounded like a MAC-10 machine pistol from the piano alcove at the north end of the room. The bullets went wild, but Larry was in a cross fire with almost no cover. The secret door closed and disappeared into the wall. Not even a seem. Those old world craftsmen were good.

Larry pointed the shot gun at the piano and fired. He worked the slide as he rolled the other direction and fire again, but he was too late. Cisco had shot the man in the leg and he was falling. The man took cover behind a large chair. The shot gun made a ragged hole in the door. Larry cocked the shot gun and fire again at the piano, but could not see a target. He needed better cover, so he scrambled to a table next to where the secret door had been. He turned it over just as a trail of bullets reached him from the MAC-10, shattering the wood of a heavy table leg.

"Cisco, Let's go!"

"No! I'm going to get us the plates. Keep them busy for a minute, that's all I need. Can you get to the front door?"

"We don't have a choice do we?"

"I'll go out the window and meet you on the road. Quit playing around and shoot to kill. These ass-holes deserve to die." Cisco disappeared through the door to the sitting room.

The man behind the piano had loaded another clip and started shooting up the table in front of Larry. A bullet penetrated the oak and scraped by Larry's left shoulder. It was only a minor flesh wound but it hurt like hell and pissed Larry off. He kicked the table away and stood aiming the shot gun at the piano. He pumped and fired until the gun was empty then he pulled the Glock and fired another three rounds into the alcove. The gunman died of multiple wounds. The man on the end of the room had been nursing his leg wound when he saw Larry stand. As he turned, Larry heard the man slam a new clip into his 9mm. He walked toward the goon and fired into the man until he quit moving.

A man appeared on the landing at the top of the stairs. Larry fired and ran for the front door. The new threat would be coming down the stairs, although he was out of sight for now. At the door Larry glanced back to the dining room. All he could see was Bruno shooting at the south end of the table. Larry went through the heavy door.

In the sitting room, Cisco sat cross-leg in front of the safe. He stretched his arms wide and took several deep breaths, emptying his mind and blocking out all the gunfire. When he felt calm and composed, he opened his eyes and smiled at the safe. His knowledge and safes came from an expensive underground book written by a master thief while in prison. It was a black market school for thieves. He had used his lock picking abilities many times, but not really being a thief, he rarely got a chance to open a safe. This was important. He just had to do it. He touched the dial and tested the drag, it moved freely to the left and stopped at a notch. If he was lucky, Bruno had not turned it past this first notch. He turned it slowly back to the right, finally, it clicked open. He was laughing in triumph as he turned the handle and the door to the safe opened. The book had said that you "didn't need to be a safecracker to open most safes, because people just were to lazy to lock them." The author was right.

Inside was a large pile of cash. He was not a robber, but this money was owed to the Flores family. It was way too much to carry now. He took one short stack of one hundred dollar bills and stuck it in his shirt, for 'bribes and expenses.' Then he lifted up the side of the large recliner and slid all the money under it. If he was lucky, it would be there later. All the plates were stacked inside, wrapped in purple velvet. Again, there were more plates than he expected and they were heavier than he imagined. Looking around the room, he spied a plastic case with a handle the size of a small suit case. It had probably contained some piece of this high tech gear they had hooked up in the room. Carefully, he placed the plates in the case and added a small sofa pillow to keep them from moving around. It was time to go. He picked up a small table and threw it through the window. As he was climbing on the ledge, the man who had come down the stairs started shooting at him. Amidst a hail of bullets, Cisco jumped the fifteen or so feet to the ground, got up and sprinted for the low wall. He made it over without a scratch.

Moving down the hill in the twilight was difficult with the heavy case. As he stepped into a clearing, a tall man dressed in fatigues stepped out from behind a large bush. The man had a high tech looking rifle pointed at him. Cisco couldn't stop his downward motion on the hillside and almost ran into the barrel of the gun.

"Stay still, do not move," the man said in Spanish, then he switched to English. "Cisco, it"s me, Trevor. We met at a restaurant once with Larry or ah, Sully."

"You don't look like Trevor!"

"It's the nose. Don't jump me, I'm on your side." Trevor lowered the gun and wiggled the false nose until it broke free of the actors paste and came off. "See, now do I look familiar?"

Cisco looked at the gun. "It must have been you who took out the two guys in the hall. What are you doing here?"

"I came to help. I had a bad feeling about this meeting."

"You are working with señor Sully?"

"Yeah, sort of, only he don't know it. I'm supposed to back him up in case he got into trouble. What's in the case? I have watched you for years and I know how honest you are, so that must be the plates to the funny money, right?"

"Sully is going to meet me on the road. We better get over there."

The pair walked around a small bluff and down onto the road just as the silver truck came around the corner. Larry slid to a stop in a choking cloud of dust, and jumped out of the four-by-four.

"Trevor! What the hell are you doing here."

"Saving your butt."

"That was you with the rifle? Why are you here? This is Mexico for Christ's sake."

"He says he's your back-up man, only your not suppose to know."

"Who do you work for?" Larry had the Glock in his hand, pointed in Trevor's direction, but not really at him. Kind of a none threatening threat.

"I work like you do. I'm a contract player for the 'Feds', just like you. Your…our contact on this case is a red headed treasury agent name Smith who is so green that they had to hire a wet nurse to wipe his nose. Your mission is to go into Mexico to find whoever was behind the new phony money that hit Seattle a few weeks back. This is really my operation. I'm the one who chose you and Fast Eddie is the one who recommended you."

"You know my uncle?"

"Know him, hell kid, we've been fishing buddies for years. I've worked on half the boarder cases that you've worked on and you didn't even know it."

"Okay." Larry holstered the gun. "This is fun but the bad guys could be coming around the corner any second."

Just then the black Mercedes roared around the preverbal corner. As it went past the pickup, Carlos casually tossed a grenade into the back of the truck.

"GRENADE!" Cisco yelled. Everybody scattered. A long thirty seconds went by, then sixty, then it was two minutes.

"What'd you think?" Trevor stood up and moved towards the vehicle. "Must be a dud."

"Be careful T."

Larry rose slowly as Trevor reached the back of the pickup and slowly put his long arm over the side. His hand came back into view with the grenade. He threw it as far as he could. They all heard it hit the ground and started to laugh from nervous release, then it exploded and showered the area with dust.

Trevor wiped his brow with a bandanna. "You know that Carlos feller is just plain mean."

The wheels in Cisco's mind clicked into a solid idea.

"YOU must have a car or something around here, right?" Trevor nodded the affirmative. "We have to go back."

"What are you talking about? We barely got out alive. By the way did you get the plates?"

Cisco walked over and picked up the now dirty case and handed it to Larry. "Here you go Señor Sullivan, or what did he call you? Larry?"

Larry looked at Trevor with a scowl.

"I'm sorry, I didn't know you hadn't told him. It just came out. Why do we have to go back, kid?"

"We left the most valuable stuff behind. Uncle Pedro and the Flores family."

"Do you know where they went? I saw them all disappear into the wall under the stair case."

"There is a tunnel that comes out in the family grave yard. It's not fair to abandon them. It's dark now. The graveyard is behind the stables."

"Okay." Larry said. "But let's not risk the plates. We'll take Trevor's ride 'cause they won't know it. One of us has to get out of here with the plates. How do we do this?"

"I'll go with the kid, you take the plates into town. You better not go to the hotel." Trevor assumed that Larry would want to stay with the plates.

"We can meet at uncle Pedro's place. He keeps a key in the drain at the end of the ally. He is sure that the Italians don't know where he lives."

Larry seemed agitated. "Wait a minute. Trevor you've had us under surveillance down here, right?"

Trevor nodded.

"So you know where Pedro lives, right?"

Another affirmative nod.

"Okay, then you take the plates and I'll go with Cisco. With out Cisco, I'm just another gringo down here, but you must have contacts. If we don't come back you can get back to the states with the plates and the information. Do you have any idea who the other dinner guest was?"

"Not really, I heard Bennette introduce them as Carlos and Mr. Wolf..... Oh my God. Was that Wolf as in the European counterfeiter "The Wolf!"

"I believe so. If we still have a chance to get him, that would be the biggest fish in this pond."

Tossing the keys to Larry, Trevor took the case and climbed into the truck.

"Be careful with the car, I borrowed it from the local CIA guys. And put this fine weapon back in the trunk, would you? It's about a hundred yards down the road in the bushes on the west side of the road."

The truck shone silver as it sped away in the moonlight. The two men walked down to the car before speaking.

The Mexican spoke first. "Can we trust him?"

"No choice. As you said, the important thing is the people we need to save. Your uncle made a big impression on me about the injustice that had fallen on the Flores family. And that was quite a stunt he pulled. Were you in on it?"

"No señor. I was just as surprised as you. I know he screwed up your plans, but maybe we can turn this into a good thing."

"Maybe double good, no, triple good. Let's go."

They drove past the hacienda slowly with the lights off. There seemed to be little going on in the courtyard. Two sets of men were moving bodies into the stables. Larry hoped that they were waiting for the morning sun to bury them. Cisco showed him where to pull over in a pasture behind an old fashion hay stack. They made their way across the open pasture with out incident. Esmerelda recognized them as they approached the tomb of Don Sancho.

"Cisco, over here! Come quickly! Your uncle has been shot."

They found the three women and Pedro under a large sprawling willow tree. A good place to keep out of sight. Cisco had thought to bring the army field medic kit from the trunk of the car, 'just in case'.

"Uncle Pedro, what are you doing here with bullets in you?"

"I am doing my job and keeping my promise to Don Roberto. I am protecting his most prized possessions."

The old man had managed to reload one of the heavy pistols, but now it was dropping from his grasp.

"You have been both brave and foolish tonight. Why didn't you wait for us to take care of things? You could have been killed."

"No matter now, my son, I think that I have been killed. However noble, I was just a spark to ignite you and your friend here into action. I knew you could do it. Just like I knew you would come back for us."

"You aren't dead yet, uncle. These wounds aren't serious, let alone fatal. I think you are more hung-over than anything else.

"How many of them did we get?"

Larry answered. "We really don't know. A few, but I think I saw Bruno shoot Al Bennette."

"Take me back, I want to spit on the Italian pig."

"We can't, they still hold the hacienda."

"What! Let's go back and finish the job."

144

"Sorry Pedro, but you're not in any shape for that."

"Promise me you will restore the hacienda to the Flores. Promise a dying old man. Avenge me Francisco, avenge me!"

Pedro passed out just as Cisco finished wrapping the wounds.

The cook, Rosa, and the two Flores women, Esmerelda and Emanuella, all looked to Cisco to see what his answer would be.

"Okay, I promise," he said. "But the old man is not dying, he is just tired and drunk."

They all hugged him, then he and Larry carried Pedro back to the car and the six of them drove back into town.

CHAPTER 14: RUN FOR THE BOARDER

Trevor backed the big pickup into the ally as far as it would go. He scrounged around and found an old tattered tarp that he threw over the hood to make the silver less noticeable. Then he decided to wait in the cantina across from the opening to the ally, where he could see if anyone came looking for Pedro. He never felt it was wrong to be cautious. The day had been exhaughsting and his emotions were shot. Over the years, with good, solid AA under his belt, he had learned how to distance himself from the triggers that lead alcoholics to drink. Self pity and anger seldom visited him, and when they did, he knew how to turn those feelings over to God. But this was a little different. He had killed people today and it hit him hard. It wasn't the first time. His was a dangerous line of work. As a cop in Del Rio, Texas, he had killed twice. Once when an interagency task force had a shoot out with drug dealers and once in an ally when the odds were four armed gang members to one scared officer. Both shootings had been declared justifiable by the department. He also had six confirmed kills as a US Marine sniper in Viet Nam. To take a life was a horrible thing to a man with a conscious. Although, you can justify it to your bosses, how do you square it with God? Trevor knew, he'd been there before.

Drink! Why would he drink over this, or anything else. Then he wondered why drinking thinking would even enter his mind. This was the start of a recognizable thought pattern. The subconscious part of his mind that wanted him to drink would start playing games with his conscious mind. First it would look for an opening like grief, anger or guilt. Then it would insert self-pity or self-loathing and start stirring the emotions into a confused state of spiritual demoralization. If an alcoholic doesn't do something about it at this stage, his unconscious mind and poor emotional state may over-rule his spiritual side and leave him no defense against the first drink. It's called alcoholism and it's a powerful force if left unchecked. He sat quietly in the back of the cantina and asked for God's forgiveness, then he forgave himself and the people who's actions brought about the deaths. He had used this technique successfully for lots of lessor matters. The next thing to do for his sobriety was to share his feelings with another person who would understand, preferably a fellow alcoholic. Being that this concerned the killings and that he was far from his regular AA buddies, Larry would have to do. He could wait for the two of them to have some time alone.

The thought occurred to him that he had better start planning their trip back to the USA. There was a pay phone on the back wall next to his booth, so he called and left a coded message for his CIA contact to call him back. Maybe they could catch a quick ride on an airplane.

Returning to his strong cup of coffee, he realized that he should be thinking about Larry's sobriety, also. The younger man would be especially vulnerable at a time like this. Trevor was quite sure that Larry had not undergone anything like this in sobriety. When Trevor had recruited Larry for this mission, he knew how little time Larry had in the program. It was just that he was a dead ringer for Tom Sullivan and Fast Eddie said he was a natural at this kind of operation.

The phone rang and Trevor grabbed it before anyone else even reacted. His cloak and dagger friend advised him to drive back to Juarez and said to keep the car with it's goodies, he wanted a new one anyway. That car had been seen around too many of the wrong places. He followed up with a few questions about Carlos and the German. His friend had a mind like a data bank and knew all the answers.

Trevor watched as Larry and Cisco pulled into the ally. He waited a few minutes to be sure they were not followed before carrying the heavy case to Pedro's tiny apartment.

The emotional atmosphere in Pedro's three room apartment was way over the edge. The women, after being held hostage for several months, were relieved and extremely grateful to their rescuers. They kept talking, and talking about it. Sliding easily from Spanish to English, Esmerelda and Emanuella had Cisco's full attention, the three of them seated at the table. They sounded excited and full of hope. Larry was sure that grief would hit them later. Maybe in a few days when they had a chance to reflect on all that they had lost.

Rosa was in the bedroom, nursing to her personal hero, Pedro, who was only semi-conscious. The cook only spoke broken English, but she had kept up a soft Spanish dialogue directed at the old man for nearly a half an hour. She had carefully removed the guns and holsters along with the bandoleers and wrapped them all in sack-cloth. She closed the curtain to the bedroom, and when she opened it a few moments later, Pedro was wearing a night shirt. The fine set of clothing was folded neatly on the dresser. As she busied herself with Pedro's care, tears of gratitude streaked down her beautifully weathered face.

It was hard for Larry to read his young Mexican partner, even in the best of circumstances. Sitting in the homemade rocker, Larry could see sympathy and horror on the kid's face as the two Flores women related their ordeal. Cisco's eyes filled with tears and occasionally one would spill unchecked to the table top. Even a hardened, street-wise tough guy can have big heart.

A few minutes ago, Trevor had come in and after a few quick pleasantries of introduction, had settled on the ancient sofa. Just like Larry, he seemed to be lost in thoughts of his own. Although both men spoke Spanish, it seemed too much effort to keep up with the conversations around them. There were other things to think about and these people all needed to handle the days events in their own way. Too much interest from the Americans might seem to be a rude intrusion. After another half-hour had passed, Trevor stretched and stood up.

"Sully, let's go find some of that good Mexican soda."

Larry nodded and followed him out the door.

"We have a lot to talk about, you and me. Let's go over to the little place across the street. We can get a booth in the back and it's all local trade. I doubt anyone will be looking for us there."

Larry looked around inside the cantina. Only a couple of drunks at the bar. The help was courteous but uninterested. They both requested Jarritos sodas at the counter and carried them to the table.

"I know, your first question is probably about the AA side of our relationship. Yes, it's true, I've got a lot of twenty-four hours behind me. That is where I met Fast Eddie. The only lie I told you was about the cop and the cowboy. I was the cop, not the cowboy in that story."

"Okay, thanks for clearing that up. It's hard to fake some sobriety stuff. That's why I was so relieved to find that Tom Sullivan was in the program. Did you really pick me because I looked like Sullivan?"

"Yep. I showed Eddie a picture of Sully and asked him if he knew anybody that looked similar who could do an undercover job for me. He just laughed and went and got your picture. I couldn't believe it. It looked like the same man. Then when I found out that you were a contract player like me, it cinched the deal."

"Why didn't you tell me?"

"They said that you liked to work alone, and Eddie said that he would get Cisco to help you. I had known of the kid for several years, but he didn't know me. There was sure to be no chance that you would offer to work with someone as obvious as Smith. And it would have been un-natural for Sully to have a partner like me without a reason, but, he would need a border guide like Cisco, so it all worked out. Don't you think?"

"I don't know about that. Everything fell apart today and I killed people. I don't want to kill people. How the hell do we kill someone and manage to stay sober? I can see myself walking over to that bar and dumping at least a fifth of rum down me. Just for starters."

"But you won't, I won't let you right now. We have work to do at the moment. If we survive the next couple of days, we can figure out if we want to get drunk or not. Don't forget that you are a cop. You are trained to kill people, or at least be ready to kill people. Right now, we need to get busy and try to stay alive."

"Yeah, I suppose that every low life in Chihuahua will be looking for us, or at least Bennette's bunch. Or, maybe it's Bruno's bunch if Bennette 'bought the farm'. I never really killed before. I've been there when it happened. You know how it is under-cover. Sometimes it just happens and there is nothing you can do about it without being dead yourself. I suppose you've had experience with pulling the trigger?"

"It's never easy and it never gets better. Some guys just let it eat them up, some learn how to deal with it. We can spend some time talking about this stuff later. We need to get those counterfeit plates back to the 'States', preferably without getting killed ourselves."

What about the German, 'The Wolf''. Interpol has been looking for him for years. This guy is so talented and successful that he can change the economy in third world countries with his funny money. If I remember, from the reports that I read, he can make almost anybody's money. And now he has made American money, the drug trade's favorite."

"I picked up those other two girls that were there in the dinning room and brought them into town. They told me that his body guard was their cousin, a local guy named Carlos. He is apparently a real pro. I checked him out. Several years as a mercenary, trained originally by the US cloak and dagger boys to do their dirty work in Central America. He has been a privateer for about six years. Bottom line: this guy has trained his whole life to take out guys just like us. Personally, I don't like the risk. We can get word to Interpol after we cross the border."

"God! I hadn't thought about those other two girls. I told them to go out the back door when the shooting started. That brings to mind our other responsibilities. The rightful owners of the hacienda, who are over there sitting in Pedro's place. What about them. Aren't they in awful danger?"

"Larry, we have a job to do, we can't fight everybody's war for them."

"I didn't expect you to be so cold."

"Sorry, I don't mean to sound that way. Let's make an escape plan first and then see what we can do, but remember that getting these plates and all the information we have back to our superiors is our mission. When I called my spook friend, he said that the airports will be covered and that Bennette had the local police in his pockets so he said to drive back. It would be the safest."

"What about a private plane?"

"No one who we could trust right now. They guy who flew me down here is over in Sinaloa right now with the DEA."

"You flew?" Larry said rhetorically. "That big silver pickup is going to be noticed. Maybe we can use the car you've got. Will that junk heap make the trip?"

"Oh yeah it'll get there, the agency man said to keep it. Best to leave the truck here and report it as stolen."

The bell over the door rang and Cisco stepped into the dim room. Larry waved from the back of the room. Cisco picked up a Carte Blanca beer from the bar on his way by. He slid into the booth and took a pull on the beer. It looked good to both Larry and Trevor. Cisco notice Larry turn away and felt a twinge of guilt, but it passed. He had lived through a hard day and deserved a beer if he wanted it..

"Well, have you two gringos figured a way out of all this mess?"

Larry turned back and finished off his citrus flavored soda. "We need your input. You are part of this operation, too."

"Count me out."

"What?"

"Count me out. I quit. I'm staying here to help these people." Cisco looked Larry directly in his eyes. "You're a good man and a good cop, but you've started something here that needs to be finished. I spent my summers here as a teenager. I know these people and I owe uncle Pedro."

"What are you going to do?"

"Don't know yet, exactly, but I'm going to get the hacienda back to the Flores family and protect young Juan Ricardo Roberto until he can run the family and the business. It's the only right thing to do."

Trevor reached across the booth and put his hand on Cisco's shoulder. "Listen, we understand. The Flores family is in good hands with you in their corner. You know how important it is for us to get those plates back to the 'States'."

"The plates that I risked my life to steal for you guys, Señor Trevor?" Cisco had slipped into his most pitiful Mexican peon role.

"Touché." Trevor leaned back and let out a whistle. "Okay, what do you want from us?"

"Just one day and maybe one trip back up the hill to the hacienda." Cisco put on his best school by smile. "And maybe that big shinny pickup, it would be too noticeable for you to drive it out of here anyway."

Larry and Trevor looked at each other. "Done!" They said in unison.

The following morning plans were made to try and retake the hacienda. Pedro was up and around contacting some of his former co-workers, looking for assistance. A few good men were rounded up. Most were farmers, however, they would look good with guns in their hands and a scowl on their faces. Only one had any experience with a gun, but Larry hoped it wouldn't matter.

By mid-day the plan was in motion. As Larry and Cisco roared up to the gate with six armed men in the back of the pickup, Trevor and Esmerelda approached through the grave yard. Emanuella and Rosa stayed with the car by the haystack. As a back up, Trevor had linked all three groups by hand held radios.

Trevor quietly moved through the headstones until he was about fifteen feet from two men trying to dig a grave by hand in the hard earth. They had leaned their AK-47 rifles against a grave marker. He shouldered the sniper rifle and quietly picked up the two guns, handing one to Esmerelda.

One of the men stopped to wipe his brow with a dirty red bandanna and caught their movement out of the corner of his eye. It was too late to react, Trevor had the drop on them.

"Buenos tardes, amigos." Trevor motioned with the gun and they climbed out of the hole.

In English, the taller of the two said, "Are you going to kill us? We are just the grave diggers, señor."

"Grave diggers don't need guns like these. Let's see how much information you can trade for your lives."

"Yes, we know what you need. 'El Cigarro has been killed. Most of the men are dead or wounded bad, and that bastard Bruno left us behind to clean up."

"How many are here now?"

"Just us two and a wounded man in the main house. One of the Italians. The others went into the city."

"All right. You can live for now. Let's go to the house. Esmerelda, call your sister on the radio and tell her to bring the car in."

Rounding the end of the stables, Trevor could smell the unmistakable smell of death coming from inside. Apparently they had moved the bodies to the horse barn. He opened the door and peered in. There were more bodies than he could count quickly.

Larry and Cisco had gained the courtyard with no resistance. After a short conversation with Trevor, Cisco posted guards and gave them instructions to fire warning shots at anybody approaching the property.

Inside they found another bad guy sitting in the kitchen at the table with a bottle of brandy, nursing a shoulder wound. Trevor pushed his prisoners into chairs.

"Okay, some one tell me what happened. And don't try that 'no comprende' routine. We all speak Spanish here. I want to know where Bruno is, how many men he has and who killed so many of your gang."

The tall one spoke after some hesitation. "The gunshots started in the house, we were told not to go in because they had enough men inside, then the driver of the limousine came around the end of the house shooting. I've never seen anything like it. He was like a hero in an American movie, everyone was shooting at him, but no one could hit him. One by one he shot all the outside guards. My cousins, my brother! He killed them all! In just a minute or two he shot everyone in the courtyard except Bruno."

"Why didn't he shoot you two?"

"We were too scared to fire, so he didn't shoot us. That's why Bruno and the others left us here. They said we were cowards."

Cisco nudged the man with his gold plated 45. "What others? You just said that Carlos killed them all."

"Not everybody. Some men were posted away from the house. Bruno has five men with him."

"Where did they go?"

"I don't know, to look for you, I guess."

"That's not good enough!" Cisco raised his weapon to strike an angry blow.

"I know." It was the wounded man whom Cisco recognized as the man from the stairs the day before. "I'll tell you, but I want a deal. I want to go home. I'm so sick of this damn place, and if you do let me go, I can guarantee that Bruno will have a short life. I saw him kill Bennette. We don't kill our boss' in Chicago. When the Dons hear of it, well, you know what they're reaction will be."

Larry had been checking the house with Esmerelda. "The house is clear. What have we learned?"

"Our Italian friend here was just about to tell us where to find Bruno." Trevor straddled a chair, sitting down backwards on it.

"Do I have a deal?"

Trevor looked from Cisco to Larry. They both nodded in turn. "Seems as though you do."

"Okay, there is a warehouse on the street that runs past the Federal Palace. I don't know the name of the street, but the warehouse has a small red sign over the door that says 'Revistas de Lobo'. It means Wolf Magazines. That's where they print the money. They would have gone there first to check on the investment, then after you guys."

"What are they driving?"

"They took the two jeeps that belong to the hacienda."

Trevor looked at Cisco. "It's your call, you are in charge of this part of the operation."

Cisco put the automatic to the Italians temple and pulled back the hammer.

"Please let me go. I have a family, I just want to go home. I told you the truth, I swear by the Virgin Mary, Mother of God."

He backed the hammer off and lowered the gun. "Okay, I believe you, take Bennette's car and head for the border. Take these two with you and don't stop in the city. We have people watching the roads. I'm going to call and tell them you are coming. If you are not across the city and on the hi-way north in forty-five minutes, I will order them to shoot to kill. ¿Comprende?"

"Yeah, we're gone. Just one thing. Who are you guys?"

"I'm the Cisco Kid, and these are my two amigos and no one is going to mess with La Familia de Flores ever again!"

The Italian stood up, too embarrassed by the wet stain on his pants to say anything more. Trevor escorted the trio out to the car. After checking the Cadillac for weapons, he sent them on they're way.

Back inside Larry sat down and had a good laugh with Cisco.

"The Cisco Kid! Do you know how corny that is?"

"Hey it worked. I just figured that he probably grew up in Chicago watching cowboy movies."

Larry just shook his head. Rosa and Emanuella joined the group in the kitchen. Cisco left the room for a minute and returned with three packets of hundred dollar bills and handed them to Larry.

"This is to insure a safe trip back. Remember what you learned on the way down here. If you have any left over, give it to Fast Eddie, we owe him. You two better get going, we're going to be fine here at Hacienda de Flores."

After all they had been through, a handshake didn't seem like enough of a goodbye, but that was all they had time for. A few minutes later, Trevor and Larry were headed back into town.

The warehouse was about twenty blocks past the Federal Palace. It was a free standing building on a corner, with thick adobe walls and small high windows. Larry and Trevor parked across the wide street. One of the hacienda's Jeeps was parked on the side street. The front door of the warehouse was open, but there was no sound or movement that they could see.

"We may not be the first visitors they've had today." Larry observed.

Trevor started the car and slowly drove down the ally next to the building. The back door was closed. Still no sign of life. He turned onto the side street and parked the car in front of a produce truck a hundred yards down the street.

"Well, we aren't going to find out anything unless we look."

Larry was uneasy about the prospect of going in there. "You're right as usual, T., but I really don't want to go in there. Let's do it by the book. Police style, you cover my back and I'll cover yours."

They checked their weapons and moved around to the front door. No sound except for the hum of a bad florescent light in the back of the room. One by one they entered covering as many angles as they could, moving from cover to cover through the large room until they were sure they were alone. There was a sort of assembly line with printing equipment, tables and clothes dryers down the center of the room. In the back there was a small office with an expensive computer filling a large desk. One of Bruno's thugs was dead at the desk, his face in his lunch. Larry looked the body over. His neck was broken along with three of the man's fingers. At the door to a filthy restroom was another of the guards. This one had an entry wound between the eyes. It looked to be about the size of a nine millimeter bullet.

"What do you think?" Trevor said at last.

"It must be Carlos, he would know where to come. My guess is he's looking for the plates and the guy at the desk probably told him that we've got them."

Larry turned and stubbed his toe on an army field pouch. He bent down and opened the flap.

"Uh-oh, do you know anything about bombs?"

Trevor turned about three shades whiter. "Only the basics. Don't touch anything and don't pick it up. Let me get over there and look at it."

He came around to the same side of the assembly line and carefully lifted the flap with a pencil. He saw the usual group of colored wires, a detonator and about five pounds of C-4 plastique. A thirty minute timer was descending through seven minutes thirty seconds.

"Yep, it's a bomb all right. A big one. I guess the question we have to ask is 'how far can we get in seven minutes?'"

"Momma said there'd be days like this."

The two men sprinted for the door and ran for the car. They were able to drive three blocks before the explosion rocked the city. They turned the car around for a drive by to look at the damage. Several neighboring buildings had broken windows but the thick walls of the warehouse contained most of the blast. The roof seemed to be gone and the interior of the building was on fire.

"So the odds are looking worse all the time. We've got Bruno with at least three thugs looking for us, and now Carlos and that Wolf fellow. Do you feel like going back to our hotels?"

"Nope! Let's just get the Hell out of town. We've got money, ammunition and gas. We could be in Juarez in four or five hours."

"Yeah, and if we're lucky, the bad guys will cancel each others tickets."

"I wouldn't count on it. But look on the bright side. Maybe Mr. Wolf will follow us to El Paso and we can grab him in the states."

Trevor headed the car for the hi-way north.

Hacienda de Flores was bustling with activity. Rosa had brought an old high backed wheel chair, the kind made from wicker, out of storage for Pedro. It was just to conserve his strength, she told him. He obliged only after he demonstrated his strength by picking her up. Then he proceeded to direct anyone who'd listen on how to clean up the mess. There were plastic sheets from the garden shed to tack over the broken windows, sharp glass to be swept up, blood stains to be scrubbed from the carpet and marble tile floors. All things belonging to the Italian devils were to be burned and much to the dismay of Pedro and Cisco, Rosa ordered all the alcohol on the premises to be dumped out. A farm tractor with a shovel attachment was brought up from the equipment barn to dig a mass grave for the dead bad guys. Cisco pointed out that if they turned the bodies over to the authorities, anything could happen. In Mexico, no bodies means no crime.

By evening the place was in presentable condition and Valentina and the children were sent for. Rosa had prepared the best meal she could on short notice, and they all sat down for a late diner.

Esmerelda sat young Juan Ricardo Roberto Flores at the head of the table. She said this was his rightful place, but that she would be in charge for him until he learned the how to handle the responsibilities. Next she proposed a toast to the 'heroes of the hacienda' and claimed that from this day forward there would be no servants at Hacienda de Flores. Everyone at the table would be considered family forever. Pedro led a prayer of thanks and the renewed family ate their first meal together. After dinner, sitting on the verandah, Esmerelda held Cisco's hand out of respect and gratitude. No words were spoken as they watched the stars and took in the cool night air.

Twenty kilometers out of Chihuahua, Larry and Trevor passed Bennette's Cadillac, smashed into a tree, full of bullet holes. It could have been Carlos or Bruno or maybe just ordinary Mexican bandits. There was no way to tell, but the two undercover agents took it as a bad sign. They traveled in silence for another hour or so until they came upon an obvious mock wreck scene.

Two four by four pickups, with roll bars and new paint jobs were at odd angles across the road. Several flares were placed in the only open path around the vehicles. As they slowed and approached the scene, Larry saw a man swing a shotgun from his shoulder, down out of sight.

"Gun!"

"Yeah, I saw it, too."

Trevor slowed as if to stop, then at the last instant he floored the gas pedal, knocking at least one man down as they slid through the opening. Larry heard several shots fired and much confused shouting. He turned to look and saw that the chase was on. Six armed men were loading into the trucks for the pursuit.

"Here they come. Now what, another shoot out?"

"Nope, those two Toyotas just don't have the power to catch us."

"What if they've put bigger motors in them?"

"It don't matter. Did you ever subscribe to 'Hot Rod' magazine when you were a kid? This old Dodge Coronet has a four hundred cubic inch V8 with two four-barrel Holly carburetors and a sweet little side-winder super charger that develops around five hundred horse power. Lean over here and look at the speedometer."

Larry looked over at the speedometer, it was a racing unit that clocked up to one hundred sixty mph, he hadn't noticed that when he had driven the car the night before.

"Are they gaining, yet?"

Yeah, slowly, but surely."

"Okay, when we get around that next corner up there, I want you to flip that unmarked switch above the ash tray."

They cleared the corner. The road ahead was straight as far as they could see. Larry hesitated until he heard a bullet glance off the roof of the Dodge. He flipped the switch and the car took off like a rocket. The sudden jump knocked Larry back so hard that he hit the head rest with a dull thud. They accelerated from eighty to one hundred thirty five in about six seconds. As the old Coronet roared across the plain, Larry just had to ask the obvious. He took a deep breath to calm himself.

"Uh… is this safe?"

"I don't know. Safer than bullets. I raced cars, as a hobby, for a while. Do you want to see how fast this baby will go?"

"No thanks."

Trevor maintained the hot cruising speed for a few minutes to be sure the bandits had given up the chase. To Larry's relief, Trevor finally reached over and turned off the switch. Back at seventy five miles per hour, the car seemed to creep along.

"How did you know it would do that?"

"Oh, I have a couple of friends over in Brownsville, Texas who build these cars for the government. Uncle Sam forks out about fifty grand for one of these ugly surveillance cars that will out perform most cop cars. Beefed up suspension, racing steering, drilled frames and always the option to go very fast. There's only one problem."

"What's that, the car turns into a pumpkin at midnight?"

"No. It uses too much gas with the supercharger on. Now we need a gas pump in the middle of nowhere."

The Dodge barely made to the out skirts of the town of El Sueco. It coughed, sputtered and quit, rolling to a stop two hundred meters from the first gas pump. Larry got out and pushed the car up to the pump while Trevor steered. Then Larry went in search of the bathroom, finding only an out house in the back. After a couple of minutes an attendant appeared and started filling the gas tank. Trevor leaned his head back and closed his eyes against the glare of the sun. Suddenly, he felt something cold and hard against the back of his neck. Slowly he put his hand up to confirm it was a gun barrel.

"¿Hable Español, gringo?"

Trevor nodded and slowly turned to see a shinny chrome 38cal. With a four inch barrel in the hand of the gas station attendant.

Speaking Spanish, the man continued. "You didn't stop to help my brother on the road. He called me to see if I could ask you why you were so rude."

"Tell him that I apologize. I thought there might have been bandits around."

"My brother thinks that you must have something important in this car to be so rude and drive away so fast."

The Mexican took an unexpected deep breath. He hadn't seen Larry leave the car and he didn't hear him creep up behind him. His first indication that there was a second man was when Larry stuck the Glock in the mans crotch.

"Tell your brother we are sorry, and that we were in too much of a hurry to get home with our grass to pay the proper toll. We just have a little grass in the car, you know, for our friends back home. How much is the usual toll for your brother?"

"Uh…uh…it is one hundred American dollars, uh… one hundred for each of you."

"And how much for you to put your gun away and fill our gas tank like a gentleman." Larry cocked the Glock.

The Mexican's hand trembled and he closed his eyes, but he lowered his gun. Then realizing that he wasn't going to loose his manhood, he answered the question.

"I should have an equal amount, Señor, for my trouble. And maybe you would like to pay me another hundred to keep my mouth shut."

Larry couldn't help but grin. "Put your gun away and let's do business."

The attendant complied. Larry laid his gun on the hood of the Dodge and counted out three one hundred dollar bills. The man reached for the money.

"Wait!" Larry picked up the Glock and pointed it at two five gallon cans against the building. "Another hundred for those two cans full of gas, deal?"

The man looked from Larry to the cans and back again with a grin. "Si Señor."

"And one more thing, if anybody asked about two gringos, you saw us driving a big silver pickup. ¿Comprende?"

For the Mexican, opportunity didn't exactly knock every day, and his brother had always told him it never hurt to ask. He wiped a greasy coverall sleeve across his face to keep from grinning again.

"Oh, Señor, you know it's much harder to remember what to say than it is to just forget you were here."

Larry pealed off another two hundred dollar bills. "You drive a hard bargain. Do you know what will happen if you go back on the deal, amigo?"

"Si Señor. You do not need to worry. We are friends now, Si?" With that he scooped up the money and hurried to fill the two extra cans.

Larry waited until the car was gassed and the two cans stored in the trunk before getting back into the car.

"Nice work, partner. Do you think we can trust him?"

"Hell no. He's probably on the phone to some cousin that lives up the road right now. But we didn't have to kill anybody this time and it was Bennette's money."

They drove to the other side of town and paid to drive up the toll road to Villa Ahumada, the last stop before Ciudad Juarez.

"I think we should dump this car and wait until dark to go into the city." Larry took a long pull on the bottle of water he picked up at the gas station.

"I was just thinking about that. I know a guy in Ahumada that would trade this car for another one. His name is Enrique Perez, everyone calls him 'Ricky'. He supplies cars and trucks for minor drug runners and border jumpers. Makes a decent living, just because he owns a big barn to store them in, and it's not illegal to sell a car."

"If you know him he's probably a snitch or something."

"Let's just say that the DEA puts money in his wife's bank account every month."

At the car barn Trevor exchanged the Dodge Coronet for a 1992 Ford Tempo. The look of a family car would help at the border. It was a deep green car with a clean interior and no outstanding features.

Ricky seemed to be in a hurry for them to leave. Trevor grabbed the car dealer by the arm.

"Hey, Ricky, we've know each other for years down here. What's the deal, amigo? No time for old friends?'

"Sorry, 'Big T.' I've got things going on. I'm glad to help you as always, but, you guys are hot. It's a high tech world you know. I got word from my sources in Juarez this afternoon. Some Italian guy has the ear of 'Groupa Diablo'. They've already got twenty thousand American on your heads. Dead or alive. And that's twenty thousand a piece."

"Damn those satellites. It's just too easy to pass the word these days. Is the Italian in the city?"

"Yeah, he got into Juarez last night. There is probably five thousand guys looking for you two. So, do me a favor and hit me over the head and take a couple of cars. If I don't report it to 'Groupa Diablo', I'm outta business. Maybe even dead. I'll wait as long as I can and forget the license plate numbers. That's the best I can do."

Larry was standing behind Ricky, so he pulled out the Glock and slapped Ricky above the left ear. Ricky went down in a heap. Trevor gave Larry a started look.

"Well, he said to do it. I always think it hurts less if you don't see it coming."

"Are you sure I was done gathering intelligence, hot shot?"

"The guy was compromised, how could we know what the truth really is after that? Come on, let's change the plates on this Green Tempo and get out of here. You can kiss and make up later."

They changed the plates and took the Tempo and headed into Ciudad Juarez. Both men were scared, but neither one wanted to talk about it. Bruno, Carlos, Mr. Wolf and now the biggest Mexican gang on the border all had it in for them. It was going to be a tense couple of days until they got across the border.

The farmhand at the hacienda gate called Cisco on one of the warlike talkies that Trevor had left.

"Señor Cisco. A big limousine is coming up the road."

"Okay, I'll be right there. Send two men around in the bushes to come up behind them. Keep the gate locked until I get there."

Carlos slowed the Mercedes to a stop thirty feet in front of the gate. He watched as Cisco and Esmerelda came through the gate, locking it behind them. There was a man on the wall on each side of the gate. Both were armed with assault rifles. Carlos checked the mirrors and saw one man cross the road behind the car while another stood off to the left about ten meters. Cisco and the woman both carried double barreled four-ten shot guns at the ready.

"You better let me handle this boss. If the Italians have gone, I'd rather not have to shoot these people. If one of them made a move towards you, I would have to kill them all."

"Do what you think is best, Carlos, we are partners from now on. All I want is the plates, If they find they're way to the United States, the American government will have an excuse to extradite me from almost any country on earth."

Carlos pulled off his sport coat and stood up out of the car with a Beretta in each hand. He stepped away from the car and pointed both guns at the dirt. It was almost dark out side, so he left the headlights on bright to claim another tiny advantage.

"Cisco, we don't have any quarrel with you. We just came for our property." Carlos sounded friendly, speaking in Spanish, like a neighbor coming to claim a lost cow. "Have the Italian devils gone?"

"Don't come any closer. This is Esmerelda Flores. She is the rightful owner of this property, the hacienda, the ranch and all you see here. La Familia de Flores has reclaimed their rights and my men are prepared to die for them. Everyone here knows how many men you killed yesterday. You are very good señor, but so am I. If you must settle your claims with violence, then put down your weapons and we can go man to man. To the death, señor."

Carlos smiled. The young rooster was trying to protect a bunch of farm hands holding guns. The kid had more guts than common sense. By making it personal, he told Carlos that his men were not up to a fight. This served to assure Carlos of a win if the shooting started. And then there was this courageous woman standing defiantly in harms way. Standing up for what was hers. Some how the whole scene touched Carlos and softened his heart.

"Listen, amigo, we are not robbers or gangsters. We were just doing business with those dogs. You are welcome to keep all that is yours, but the plates belong to Señor Lobo. If the Italians have been beaten by you and your strong army, you have no need for our property. We will even buy them from you. What do you say. No one has to get hurt here."

Cisco felt fate skip a beat. Maybe he would live through this encounter and at the same time have a chance to send a big prize to his friends, Larry and Trevor.

159

"The Italian dogs took your property with them when they fled the hacienda. The safe where we both saw them stored was empty when we took the house."

"Do you know where they have gone? Is Al Bennette still alive?"

"They have gone after Sully. They blame him for what happened here yesterday. Bruno is in charge and Bennette is dead. I spit on his grave myself this afternoon. I think they went for the border. Probably Ciudad Juárez."

"Then why, may I ask, are you still here?"

"These are my people, I spent many summers here as a boy. They need my help." Do you understand that kind of loyalty?"

Carlos holstered one gun and put the other in his waste band. He stepped up to Esmerelda's shotgun. She pulled back the hammers for both barrels but didn't flinch. No shaking, no sweating, no fear. He believed she would shoot without hesitation. He found it sad that such a beautiful woman should be so cold and willing to kill. She must have suffered much at the hands of the Italians.

"Vía con Dios, Señora." He smiled warmly and turned away.

Von Stein lit his pipe as Carlos drove back down the road. He was a thinker, and this all needed some planning.

"Carlos, call home and have Garcia fly the helicopter to El Paso."

"Don't you wish to go with him, Señor?"

"No. I don't want to take a chance on the DEA or some other organization running down the flight and finding me as a prize. Have him file a normal flight plan to El Paso air park for maintenance. And drive us to Juarez as quickly as possible."

The phone call was made as they crossed the city. Von Stein leaned back and closed his eyes as the big car sped northward on the blacktop.

CHAPTER 15: HIDE AND SEEK

The pay phone was in the back of Chihuahua Charlie's' Restaurant on the Plaza de Americas in downtown Juarez. Trevor tried to make sure no one was paying any attention to him as he dialed. The restaurant, always a popular spot with the tourists, was exceptionally busy with the late dinner crowd. This made Trevor a bit nervous about discovery, however he had been a player on the border long enough to know how to blend in. The knowledge that most people are too concerned with themselves to notice a stranger was small comfort when your life could depend on anonymity, but contact with the 'FEDS' was important. He had tried dialing the Treasury office in El Paso, but of coarse it was too late for anybody to be working. Then he tried to contact Jerry Smith, the red-headed special agent, at home, but the number was disconnected. That was a very bad sign. Smith was the contact man for this operation and the only person of authority that Trevor had dealt with on this assignment. Trevor knew that Smith was a real agent, he had checked him out independently, using his contacts at the FBI. Working undercover meant that you always had to be sure of whom you deal with, especially in the US Government. Too many bureaucracies with too many operations going on, each unaware of the other. Just as Jerry Smiths' cell phone reported an 'out of service' message, Larry came out of the rest-room room close by.

"Any luck? Larry tried to be as casual as possible.

"No good. All the numbers I have for Smith are disconnected or not working.

"Let me try, I made him use a different cell phone." Larry took the telephone and dialed the number of the special cell phone he and Smith had set up. It was out of service, also.

"Well, why don't we just drive over there and go to the city police station. They'll have the numbers for the red-head or his boss." As soon as Larry said it, he knew why. Big city police stations leak like a fisherman's net. Court reporters and paid informants reside in almost every metropolitan police station. If their cover was blown at this time, they would surely die.

"You don't really think that's a good idea, do you?"

"Naw, why don't we call Fast Eddie and see if he can get us across and safe."

Larry made the call and talked for several minutes while Trevor sat back at a near by table, smoking a cigarette. When Larry sat down he put it out.

"I didn't realized that you smoked."

"Really? Well that's about the tenth one I've smoked today, and you've been with me all day."

"I must be getting senile. I didn't even notice, and I'm one of those reformed non-smokers that everyone complains about."

"What did the hamburger king have to say?

"He said the same thing that your car salesman said, that we are too hot to cross the border here. The Mexicans are watching for us at the border for Groupa Diablo on this side and Italians from up north are showing up to grab us on the El Paso side. The 'Feds' can't do anything as long as we are on this side and you know that the Mexican Federales are in the hip pocket of Don Alonso and El Gordo."

"Did he have any news about Jerry Smith?"

"Yeah, that red headed peacock was arrested by the internal affairs guys about the same time that we went to Ciudad Chihuahua. I guess he was a habitual gambler and had been stealing evidence money all over the place. He was my only contact on this case and if he was your only contact, then we are screwed until we can get back to the world where someone knows who we are."

"Who is your assignment man?"

"It's my old captain from when I was a patrol officer, Captain Moffitt in Albuquerque."

"Wow, that's where my assignments come from, too. I guess, we go to Albuquerque, if we can get across the damn border. Is Eddie going to help us?"

"He said that with Cisco out of town, his resources are limited and that we are just too hot to cross here at El Paso. Also, not to trust any authorities right now, on either side of the border. Too much greed being fed by way to much money around here. Eddy's suggestion was to get out of Juarez, without getting killed, and do an illegal crossing somewhere close by."

"Did he say anything about Albuquerque?"

"Yep, it's our best bet, but no airports and try to stay off the interstate. He volunteered to call Moffitt, but the Captain can't do much until we are on his turf."

Larry looked up from the conversation and went pale.

"We got trouble. That big goon that guards Don Alonso just came through the door with three other guys. They're sweeping the room, looking for someone. Guess who?"

One of the men spotted the two cowboys in the back and signaled to the others. They started to converge on Larry and Trevor from different locations, but the restaurant was crowded and it was difficult to move quickly through the throngs of tourists eating, waiting and taking pictures.

Just then, an attractive Mexican woman, wearing a waitress costume, approached Larry from behind.

"¿Señor Sully?" Larry nodded, not wanting to take his eyes off of the approaching doom. "Seniors, you must come with me. Pronto."

Their options were limited and a gun battle seemed probable. Not a pretty thought in a place as confined and crowded as this. Larry finally turned to the woman. Her gaze was fixed on the approaching goons and her jaw was set in a hard line.

It was Maria, the cousin of Cisco who operated the drink carts in the market places. "Maria?"

"Si, Señor. Por favor, we must go now!"

The woman led them through a door into the kitchen and then through a maze of cramped hallways, across an alley, through a closed market center with a hundred little booths and through another maze of hallways to a tiny sleeping room.

She went to the dresser and pulled out a large drawer and set it on the bed. It contained men's clothing and stage make up and shaving items. Straw peasant hats topped the dresser.

"Cisco called me and said to watch for you. Change your appearance and go to Paquimè. There is help there." Maria turned and was gone before the two men could respond.

Trevor held up several pieces of clothing until he found a shirt and vest that would fit. Meanwhile, Larry went to the basin and shaved off his beard. It isn't easy to shave a beard when you are in a hurry, but he managed to get through it with only two or three cuts on his face. He left a healthy specimen of a mustache, hoping it would help him look more Mexican from a distance.

After dressing, the two undercover agents left the room. Each of them carried a backpack with them containing half of the money plates. They thought it was best to keep the two halves of each bill separate in case one of them was captured or somehow lost control of his backpack. They wandered the maze until they found an outside door.

The door led to a large alley, or maybe it was a small street. As they were getting their bearings, an old nineteen fifties model pickup with a tarped back roared up to them belching black smoke and knocking quite loudly. Larry put his hand in his jacket and switched the Glock 9mm safety to the off position.

"Hey Señors, this taxi is going to the ruins at Paquimè. The ride is five dollars. Do you have five dollars, Señors?"

The driver had on a ripped dirty T-shirt and smelled of garlic, but his toothless grin was disarming.

"Hola, amigo. Si, we have the money for the fare. Can we go now?"

"Si Señor Sully, it's not like the truck you gave me and my mother a ride in, but it will get us to Paquimè." The man wore a large grin.

Larry climbed into the cab and Trevor climbed into the back. Larry felt a soft squeeze on his leg and turned to see the same old Mexican-Indian woman who had sat next to him on his last trip to the ruins. She giggled and spat snooze into a paper drink cup. Larry smiled at the wonder of how these events could be brought to into place. The old woman slapped his leg hard and giggled some more as the truck lurched into gear and headed out of town.

At Paquimè the midnight moon was full over the Indian ruins and all of Larry's senses were working overtime. It had been a dangerous day and a long day, but he was not tired. He acknowledged only the feelings that led to self-preservation. A healthy dose of fear was the motivation and experience with dangerous situations, gave him the self-reliance to take any action he needed to save his life.

The driver pulled the noisy truck between two ancient crumbling walls. Someone in the distance flashed their car lights, an obvious signal. The driver stopped the truck and turned off the lights and just then, a whole appeared in the windshield, spidering outward as the sound of the report reached Larry's ears. If the grand-motherly figure next to him had been a normal size person, she would be dead, but she was unusually short, and lucky.

"It's a trap!" Larry heard Trevor's voice, but it came from the side not the back of the truck where he had been riding.

"Stay down and get out of here as soon as you can." As he said this to the driver, Larry slipped down from the seat, out the door and over the nearest low wall. The Driver started the pickup and backed slowly away. Several shots ricochet off the heavy Detroit steel.

"I'm right behind you, don't shoot me." Trevor scrambled up beside Larry, next to the wall. "I slipped off the back of the truck just as he made that last turn."

"What have you got in mind?" Trevor took a deep breath. "Looks like it's time for a strong offense. I don't think they have a starlight scope. They'll be looking for us in the ruins, let's just get back in the alley, stay in the shadows and go straight at them. I don't think they'll expect that. Maybe we can get to that car and bring the rest of them in to us."

"What were you, a Marine or something? That sounds pretty damn gung-ho to me."

"Simper Fi. Just trust me, and don't shoot unless you are going to hit something. This ain't TV. We'll run out of bullets real fast here."

"Hey T., I can shoot and count, don't worry about me. Let's go get'em before my nerve runs out."

They both went over the wall slowly and both stayed on the same side of the alley, in the shadows. Larry stayed about thirty feet behind Trevor. Just as Trevor passed an out-cropping of wall, next to a doorway, a dark figure appeared behind him from the door and raised a gun. Larry was there in an instant and hit the man with the Glock as hard as he could above the left ear. The composite/plastic gun was comparatively light, so Larry had to swing extra hard for the effect, however, it was a successful motion. The man dropped without resistance onto the sand.

Trevor heard the thud of the gun against the man's skull, but just kept going. He figured he was either dead or not dead, no time to stop and keep score. Moving targets are the hardest to hit in the dark.

As they worked their way down to the car, they began to see two people in the moonlight. A thin man with a chrome plated gun paced back and forth in front of a Corvette while a woman was apparently hand-cuffed to the bumper guard.

The woman was Maria, still in the waitress skirt and peasant blouse uniform, the man was Ricardo, her sometimes boyfriend and the gun was a .357 revolver. When they were in shooting range, Larry huddled up with Trevor.

"Did the guy you took down have a rifle? There has to be someone with a rifle somewhere."

"No he just had this forty-five." He showed him the automatic.

"The first shots were from an AK47. So we have at least two to deal with. I'll creep in closer, you watch that guy by the 'Vette, if he sees, me shoot him, but try to wait 'til the last second."

He moved on down the wall in the shadows. Larry thought it was amazing how agile the big cowboy was for a man in his sixties. Trevor was close now, maybe fifteen feet, Larry was thinking that he himself could never have gotten so close undetected when a rock exploded above Trevor's head. Ricardo was not the shooter. Then another bullet hit next to Larry's face, throwing rock chips and sand into his face. He felt the blood start to run out of his cheek from a superficial cut. He flattened out instantly. It was his job to watch his partner's back, but it was too late. When he looked up Trevor was lunging at Ricardo just as Ricardo raised his revolver to shoot. Larry had landed with his own gun under him and the newly acquired forty-five was stuck in his belt. He was helpless to make any difference in Trevor's situation.

Ricardo fired at Trevor's head from point blank range and missed, the heavy gun was too hard to control at arms length. Too bad for Ricardo. Trevor slammed his fist into Ricardo's throat at the Adams-apple. With his other hand he reached down and pulled up Ricardo's knee, throwing him off balance and over backward. As Ricardo fell, Trevor wrenched the pistol from his grasp. He turned the gun around to shoot, it wasn't needed. Ricardo had hit his head on the car as he went down. Trevor knew that being unconscious with a throat swelling shut from the harsh blow, Ricardo would not survive.

Larry rolled across the ground to the opposite wall, trying to get out of the line of fire. He saw that the move was a correct one when the rifleman put two more shots into Larry's old position. Larry got up and ran down to the car, aware that he was exposed in the moonlight. Trevor was searching Ricardo's pockets for the key to Maria's handcuffs.

"How many more men?" He said to the frightened woman.

"Ricardo and two others, one has an assault rifle.

The big cowboy found the keys and handed them to Larry.

"Why are you here, Maria?"

"I am suppose to get you to Guadalupe where a man named José Morales is waiting to take a group across the Rio Grande. He has a milk truck that has a compartment for six people. It's a thousand dollars each, but he has never been caught. He can't be late. He crosses the border at 4:30AM every day to sell his milk in El Paso. We must go now to have time. It must be after two by now.

"Larry looked at his watch. "Almost 2:30. Do you have a car?"

"Let's take this one. That scum-pig Ricardo don't need it."

"The handcuffs finally came loose and as Maria stood up, a bullet hit her and knocked her back against the hood of the Stingray. Trevor and Larry both turned in the direction of the shot and fired several times. No one returned their volley. Larry turned back to Maria. She just had time to say 'go', then she died. Larry was suddenly struck by the finality of death. They were having a conversation one minute, then she was gone, never to converse again. He turned to see Trevor walking up the alley as if he was crossing the street. Larry cried for a few seconds. He closed Maria's eyes and laid her on the ground. Trevor was coming back.

"We got him partner. What a shame. Maria was a good woman. I knew a lot about her, she was a border rat like me."

"Do you think we can trust what she said?"

"Yeah, she was Cisco's cousin, I think she was on our side."

"How far to Guadalupe from here?"

"About eighty miles, but I know some short cuts and we have a Corvette."

"What about Maria. Are we just going to leave her?"

"No choice. Her friends aren't far. They will take care of her. Let's go, Larry. We can't afford to miss that truck."

After sliding the seat back as far as it would go, Trevor folded himself into the sports car and told Larry to buckle up. The trip to Guadalupe was fast and dusty as half of it was on Mexican hard tack roads composed of rock and dirt packed by centuries of use. Larry did manage to fall asleep for the last twenty miles as the corvette screamed down Mexico's Hi-way 2.

In Guadalupe They spied the milk truck at a diner on the hi-way. José came out after a while picking his teeth and looking around. Larry got out and approached him.

"Hola, amigo."

José held up a hand to halt Larry's greeting. "I know who you are and what you want. Do you have the cash?"

"Sure." They stepped over into the shadow of the truck. Larry pulled two thousand out of his shirt and gave it to the man. "You're English is very good."

166

"Should be, I was born in Idaho. I just look Mexican. It's my fathers fault. He was born in Mexico City." José had an infectious warm smile. No wonder the border patrol left him alone. "Meet me behind the diner, I'll pull the truck around."

The agents walked to the back of the building. José brought the truck around but didn't stop, he drove it up to a warehouse looking building and sounded the horn. A big door slid open and he drove the truck inside. Larry and Trevor followed.

Inside there were two identical trucks. José explained that one was normal and one had the hidden compartment. Four or Five times a month he used the 'mule' truck, the rest of the time, he used the real truck. Actually, he had been stopped and searched several times, but always with the real milk truck. He would deliberately act suspicious and the stupid border guards would fall for it and search his rig, only to find milk. On the average, they came to know him as a regular and left him alone. He played his little game on all new patrol agents, however tonight would be a cinch. An old friend of his was on the gate at the bridge.

The rear of the large stainless steel cylinder on the back of the truck opened up and they squeezed onto the benches with four Mexican men. The crossing into the United States was as José said it would be, and he let them out close to the rest area on Interstate 10, east of El Paso. At the rest area they changed back into gringo clothes and after a couple hours they were able to hitch a ride with a minister and his wife in a Winnebago. They gave the nice couple the story that they were robbed in Mexico and barely made it out alive. The couple drove them straight through to Las Cruces as Larry and Trevor sat at the small dinette in the motor home.. They were dropped off a few blocks from the storage place where he had the silver mini-van stashed, the one he had driven down from Albuquerque.

"I've got a car stashed close, over there on the next block I'm really burnt to a crisp, we need some rest. That's another thing about cops on TV, they never have to rest unless there's a beautiful woman involved. I felt reasonably secure at the City Center Motel."

"That's a good place, but we are both known there and me, well, let's just say that I've been in most of the rooms over the years. Why don't we drive over the mountains to Alamogordo. We'd be taking the long way around to Albuquerque and the roads offer us several options from there."

"It's been a tough couple of days, but I guess I can stay awake for the next couple of hours."

"Just cowboy up! We'll be there in no time."

After retrieving the van, Larry stopped by Ralph's Gun's for more ammo, just in case, and then proceeded towards the Organ Mountains and the New

Mexico's famous 'White Sands' beyond. Trevor was asleep in the passenger seat before they got out of Las Cruces. Even as tired as he was, Larry enjoyed the quiet time to think. The events of the last couple of days were just a blur. He needed to mentally sort things out and file them away in his mind. When it came to putting all this down in a report, he didn't want the facts to be confused or jumbled together.

As Larry's mind wandered through the many different events of the past few days, he started to cry, then held it in check. He was feeling things that he hadn't felt since he was a child. It was overwhelming. Fear had always played a big part in his job, but now he was more afraid of the person he was than of getting shot. He didn't want to play this game anymore. Of that he was sure, however, he and Trevor were trapped by circumstances that were way out of control. Even when he was a macho, drunken cop, he didn't want to kill anyone, and now he had. More than once, and it wasn't over yet. They were still a couple hundred miles from safety, with most of the bad guys in the state of New Mexico looking for them.

Besides fear, there was anger. He was angry at the situation and angry at himself for the things he had done. The latter led to self-loathing, and then to self-pity, but something his sponsor, Bob, had said popped into his mind.

"Alcoholics just want someone to hold them while they beat themselves up. Get off the pity pot and quit feeling sorry for yourself." He could almost here Bob's voice.

Looking over at Trevor, he wished he was awake. He could use some of his wisdom and support. Trevor was out like a light. Probably hadn't slept in three days. Larry didn't have the heart to wake him. He drove on in the morning sun, keeping himself awake by reciting affirmations and the two prayers that he could remember. The Serenity Prayer and the Lords Prayer.

The Alamo Inn is close to the railroad tracks on Hi-way 54, about in the middle of the hi-way business route for Alamogordo. Larry chuckled when he rented a room under the alias of Smith and Jones. He woke Trevor up long enough for them to gobble a couple of breakfast burritos from a take out, then they both crashed on their respective beds, fully clothed and guns close by.

It was dark when Larry awoke suddenly as if he had heard a shot. It took him a few seconds to pull reality around him like a blanket. As the world came into focus, he realized the lights were off and Trevor was standing next to the window holding his gun down by his side. He turned slowly from the window as Larry reached for the light switch.

"I wouldn't do that, chief. Looks like we're gonna have company."

"How soon?"

"I think we have a few minutes."

Larry stood up and chambered a round in the Glock. He grabbed the plastic bag with ammunition in it. He checked the forty-five that he had taken from the thug at the ruins. It was only half full, so he filled it. He had two extra clips for the Glock, so he filled them, then dumped the rest of the ammo in the back pack with the plates. He slipped on the back pack.

"I guess I'm ready, you need any bullets, T."

"No I took care of my piece while you were sleeping."

"What's happening out there?"

"Over at the restaurant I see a Jeep that looks like the ones from the hacienda and two Cadillacs next to it. Bruno and another guy went into our motel office, but they haven't come out yet."

"Is there men in the cars?"

"No they're probably eating. My guess is that they have been checking all the motels with our descriptions, probably posing as FBI or something."

"Well, they're about to hit pay dirt. That desk jockey in the office didn't look like a stand up guy to me. They can probably buy a key to our room for twenty bucks. I say we jump in the van and high tail it out of Dodge before they get organized."

"I'm for that, but we need to go out the bathroom window. I moved the van next door while you were asleep."

The bathroom window was large and low, so it wasn't too much trouble for the agents to slip out that back. The only problem was that they were trapped between two buildings in sort of an alley about five feet wide. They were about fifty feet from the exit to the street when a man's silhouette appeared at the end of the alley with a shotgun. The man fired as soon as he saw them. Larry saw chunks of plaster fly off the wall in front of them. They back peddled a few steps then turned and ran back up the alley. Another man was coming through the bathroom window that they had just left. They were definitely trapped.

"Give me your foot!"

Trevor made a step with his hands. Larry instantly understood and put his foot in Trevor's clasped hands. Trevor almost threw Larry onto the roof of the motel, then he threw his back pack up and jumped for the roof line. Because of his height, long arms and the low adobe style building, he was able to hook an arm over the top. Larry helped him scramble up just in time. The shotgun thundered again and the left heel of Trevor's cowboy boot disappeared.

On most adobe style buildings the walls are higher than the roofs. This building offered only about a foot of protection, but the men in the alley couldn't get far enough back to see the two men running across the roofs and the men on the other side didn't know where to look yet. Larry and Trevor made the far end of the building by the train tracks and let them selves down over the edge. It was a higher wall on this side so it was about a six foot drop.

Larry understood Trevor's apparent talent for the tactical side of the job. "What now, T.? You're better at this than I am."

After a quick look at the terrain, Trevor answered. "Our best plan is to let them come to us and take care of it. Maybe the locals will show up, but if they do we have to have a back door."

"We don't even know how many. How do we win against odds like ten to two, or what ever it is."

"Well, we set up a kill zone and make enough noise for the cops to get involved, then while they are arresting the bad guys, we sneak out the back. Now listen, the van is parked at the next motel to the south of the one we were in. The door is unlocked and the key is under the passenger seat. I'm going to be up on that signal tower over there and you set up in that box car back there. The furthest one. They'll come from both sides of the buildings. When you see them close together, take out that forty-five and blast away. You don't have to hit anyone, just draw them towards you. When the gun is empty, jump out the back side of the box car and sneak toward the south. Try to get to the van and bring it down the main hi-way past the restaurant and wait for me. I'll be there."

"What are you going to do!"

"What I trained for, hopefully, I'll buy us enough time to get to Albuquerque. Now go, and remember, sneak, don't run. Go slow when you leave that box car."

With that Larry headed to the waiting train. Trevor walked over to a railroad workers pickup and smashed the side window with his handgun. In the glove box, he found a box of 30-30 ammo that matched the Remington rifle in the gun rack. In the tool box he found a short length of rope. Then he climbed the tower and secured the rope so that he could use it for a fast get away. He settled in a sitting position on top of the signal box. He didn't have any cover, but his plan was to get three to five shots off and be gone.

A few seconds later he saw two men coming from the north side, moving slow and cautious. Both carried full size shotguns. A shadow on the southern most building showed three more figures moving through the rail yard. The two groups were a hundred yards apart and moving closer to each other with every second. Trevor prayed for Larry to wait a couple of minutes.

When the two groups of thugs were about fifty feet apart, one of the men made a call on a cellular phone. A moment later, one of the Cadillacs rounded the corner from the north and drove along the tracks to the stalkers. When it stopped, five more men got out, one of them was Bruno. While the first men were dressed in jeans and light jackets, these men were dressed in suits-even Bruno.

Trevor took aim on the furthest man, intending to shoot him in the leg. He waited for Larry to make his move, and soon enough, a hail of bullets came from the box car. All the men turned away from Trevor's position and started moving Larry's direction. Just as Trevor pulled the trigger, the head of a man moved into

170

his line of fire. It was Bruno, who was much closer to his position. It was too late to stop the action, Bruno fell, instantly dead with the bullet entering just above the right ear.

None of the men saw where the rifle shot came from. They were yelling about it, being Bruno, and that he was dead. Trevor slowly worked the bolt action, loading a round and holding two more cartridges between his fingers for a fast reload. He waited until they started moving again. This time, they were more aggressive, obviously mad about Bruno. Trevor took a deep breath and let it out slow, squeezing off another round at the end of the breath. An Italian took the round in the right leg. Trevor breathed again as he quickly loaded another bullet and repeated the action, another thug fell. Four seconds later one more bad guy went down screaming in pain.

The group now knew his position, so Trevor grabbed the rope and slid down, leaving the rifle on the signal box. He ran full out to the pickup where he had stolen the Remington. He didn't look back to see, but none of the men immediately followed him. He threw open the door of the Chevy and jerked the wires down from the dash. Quickly he twisted two wires together and touched a third to the twisted pair as he pumped the gas pedal. The truck roared to life. He slammed it into gear and spun the tires in the gravel, drove down the railway tracks, turned down the side of the motel and left the pickup at the restaurant. He crossed the hi-way on foot and waited in the shadows of a closed tire shop. Sirens were coming from all directions. He hoped Larry had got away clean. He had to trust that Larry was a professional and could keep his head. Panic can get you killed in this business. Presently the mini-van came down the street and pulled over to let several police cars converge on the railway. Trevor walked calmly from the shadows as if Larry was picking him up to go bowling. As the city police, sheriffs deputies and state troopers all headed to the backside of the motel, the two men with the multi-million dollar backpacks headed north on HI-way 54.

Lieth Von Stein and Carlos were in the air over Las Cruces monitoring police channels when they heard about the Alamogordo gunfight over the state police band. Having had a few minutes of quality time with Bruno's men at the counterfeiting shop and again when they found Bennette's Cadillac speeding out of Ciudad Chihuahua, They surmised that Sully had the plates. Another good guess was that Sully would go to the USA. A third correct guess was that Bruno and his Mafia connections would have the man power to flush Tom Sullivan out. After a few minutes the police reported that two men in a silver mini-van headed north and were wanted for questioning about the gunfight. Von Stein spoke to his helicopter pilot over the helmet intercom.

"Fly us straight to Alamogordo, pronto."

"No can do, boss. White Sands missile range is between here and Alamogordo."

"Well, how big is it?"

"The range runs about a hundred and forty miles in length. If we try to cross it, they'll scramble F-14 jets from Biggs Air Base and could even shoot us down."

"Can't we go around it down by El Paso?"

"No. Fort Bliss is a no fly zone also, and we can't cross the border without a flight plan or the DEA will get us for sure. The only place we could go around would be at the airport, but we may have to wait two hours for clearance to cross the commercial flight lanes."

"Okay, he is probably moving north to Albuquerque anyway. Probably to catch a flight to New York or Los Angeles, where he can sell the plates. Or maybe he'll sell them to the police."

Carlos joined in. "I think he wants to use the plates, but we can't risk anybody finding them in the United States."

"Well boss, if we have to fly around White Sands, they have to drive around it. Let's go to the airport so I can get more fuel for this bird and something to eat. This baby will get us to the other end of White Sans in about twenty-five minutes."

Seven minutes later, at the El Paso International Airport, they were tying down the McDonald Douglas model 520 helicopter. It was a midnight blue beauty with silver pin-striping and a fox gray interior that sat four, including the pilot, who was on his way to the airport diner for take out.

"So who do you think the second man is."

"I'm not sure, but as I remember the events at Bennette's house, it seems like at least one shot, or maybe two came from out side of the house. Out the back, and now that I think about it those shots must have been rifle fire from a good distance, because I don't remember hearing the report instantly."

"So, this Sullivan character must have had a back up shooter."

"That solves the second man mystery, but something else has been bothering me. If Sully is Mafia, then why are the Mafia trying to kill him."

"That's easy. Bruno told them that Sully killed Bennette."

"But didn't you say you saw Bruno shoot Bennette? Why wouldn't he just go and clear his name with the bosses? And how would he know that Bruno told them that?"

"Good question, could be he has gone solo, or maybe he is a policeman of some sort. Let's go see if there is somewhere around here to get my laptop online. Maybe we can get a line on this silver van. Maybe the police have a license plate number or something."

CHAPTER 16: LOST AND FOUND

It was the dark blue, metal flake paint job that somehow made the car look extremely fast. The fact was, that it really was very fast. A nineteen sixty four Pontiac GTO, commonly called a 'goat', with a souped up motor and suspension. But it wasn't just the speed and the looks that attracted him to the car, it was a big car made heavy with real steel. The kind of fine ride that just isn't made anymore. On the front seat, next to the sawed off shot gun and a CAR-15 assault weapon, was a large bucket of fried chicken. The one thing he missed most in prison was good fried chicken. He could eat it hot, he could eat it cold, and he could even eat it three days old. He had picked this bucket of foul up late last night as he left Los Lunas and expected the chicken, along with his two fifths of Jack Daniels whiskey to last until noon.

The sun was just coming up in the desert. That was another thing that he missed in the Colorado state prison. He always liked to watch the sun come up before he went to bed. Being forced to reverse his nocturnal schedule make lock up hell for Bumper Blue. That all changed eleven days earlier when he had overpowered and killed the two guards who were driving him to Santa Fe to stand trial for his crimes in New Mexico. It was bad enough that they convicted him of trafficking in Colorado, but they wanted him for murder and distribution of a controlled substance in New Mexico, and in Texas they had a whole list of charges from racketeering to kidnapping. All of this because of that punk cop Larry. Of course, he knew the dude as Manny Grant. He didn't find out his real name until the undercover cop's affidavit was read during his trial. After his escape it didn't take long to plug back in to his old contacts, including his shirt-tailed Mafia connections around Albuquerque. He found out that this Larry Kelly guy was working undercover around the Mexican border. Then when he got news that the Mafia, and nearly everyone else was looking for a guy headed north who might be a cop, he figured it must be the same guy. Why not. If it wasn't, well, at least he might find a place to vent some of his revenge.

The brand new police band scanner that hung under the dashboard had been donated to the cause by a Bernalillio County Deputy Sheriff who had the misfortune of stopping Bumper on a deserted back road south of Albuquerque. He had left the deputy inside his burning patrol car at the bottom of a ravine. The police scanner was a great thing to have. It told him all he needed to know, and now he was sitting here waiting for a silver mini-van to come by. Easy work for man who considered himself, quite proudly, to be a master criminal.

The little town of Mountainair sits at the junction of New Mexico Hi-ways 55 and 60. Bumper chose this location to wait because it was on the route of several back-road ways into the big city. He assumed that anyone smart enough to infiltrate his gang, would know enough to stay off the free-way. If he were driving north from Alamogordo, he could come into Mountainair from three different routes and leave by just as many. All roads from this point could lead to Albuquerque. The path up Interstate 25 didn't seem likely and the other way, going through the town of Vaughn and up to Interstate 40 would be too far out of the way. The mini-van would come this way, Bumper was sure of it. However, for the time being, he had his whiskey, chicken and a police scanner. Sitting in this fine stolen car, plotting Larry's demise, was about as sweet as it could get, for Bumper Blue. Every so often he needed to re-enforce the Jack Daniels with a line of cocaine, just to keep his edge.

Jackie swung her feet over the edge of the bed at three forty-five AM, it was an act of defeat. She had been laying awake for the past hour or so. Something just didn't feel right in her world. It was hard to put her finger on it, or put a name to it, or put a face on it. Something was just wrong, or, something was going to go wrong. Her usual rising time was four o'clock and ever since she had made the decision to join the 'Double B' team on the Lifeguard helicopter, as a full time flight nurse, she had been eager to get up and go to work. Every day seemed to be one adventure after another. The guys were great to work with. Brian Green, the co-pilot and paramedic had a real funny bone-humor that is important when you see the worst of tragedies day in and day out. The other Brian, Brian Paterson, was always the serious professional and his ability to fly the aircraft was uncanny. The other pilots at Lifeguard all said he was the best they had ever seen. Jackie thought he was cute behind those mirrored sunglasses, but he was a happily married man.

She did her morning ritual, the Serenity Prayer, The Lords Prayer and the Seventh Step Prayer. It was the last prayer that gave her the most strength. 'God, I am now willing that you should have all of me, good and bad. I pray that you now remove from me every single defect of character which stands in the way of my usefulness to you and my fellows. Grant me strength, as I go out from here to do your bidding. Amen.' After her daily dose of spiritual closeness with her higher power, she was usually ready for the day, but not today. Her emotions were running amuck in a wind storm of doubt and loathing.

After forcing herself to take a shower, get dressed and drink a cup of coffee, she drove to the airfield. She was early, so she just sat in her car for a while drinking coffee out of a thermos cup, watching the sky go from pitch black to steel gray. Brian, the pilot was at the helicopter doing preflight stuff. No matter how early she was, he was always there first. She looked over to the Sandia Mountains where the sun would soon rise. When she looked back, Brian Paterson was at her window.

"You okay this morning, Jackie?"

She gathered her things and opened the car door. "Sure, Brian, I'm all right. Just didn't sleep well, I guess."

"You look like you had bad news or something. You know the way people look when we have to tell them that a loved one has passed."

"That bad, huh."

"It was a full moon last night. I'm sure it's going to be a killer day. First of the month paychecks and a full moon usually means a lot of decent folks went out and screwed up their lives last night. Do you want me to call the relief nurse?"

"No. It's nothing, really. I just need some more coffee. I'll be fine. Have I ever let you down?"

"Absolutely not. Jackie, you are the best flight nurse we've seen in a couple of years. That's why Brian and I wanted you on our team. We know that we make a real difference out there. And you get the job done, every time. No complaints from me, just concerned. That's all."

"Thanks Brian, I'm fine. Really."

As the pair walked to the ready room, Brian Green came out to meet them.

"Hi guys. We've got work already this morning. Traffic accident down by Ruidoso last night. They took a woman to the local clinic with a punctured lung and a broken back. They've got her stabilized but they want to get her up here to University Hospital where they can do more for her."

"Well let's get suited up, Ruidoso is about an hour out."

At Tularosa, Larry pulled into the all night gas station for a fill up. Trevor went next door to the café for a couple of quick sandwiches to go. As he was walking out he overheard a State Trooper's radio give a report that two men in a silver mini-van were wanted for questioning. The trooper, who was sitting at the counter reached down and turned his radio up. Just then another call came in. It was a bad car wreck up by Ruidoso. The trooper grabbed his hat and told the waitress to save his ticket and ran out the door, jumped into his cruiser and sped off. Trevor shook his head.

"Thank you God!" He said, then immediately felt guilty because the poor crash victims were providing for his temporary freedom with their misery.

When Trevor returned to the van, he instructed Larry to drive north on Hi-way 54. After a few minutes, Larry pulled over at a hi-way maintenance turn around and parked behind a gravel pile. They broke out the sandwiches.

"We're lucky guys tonight, my friend. They have us on the police radio, wanted for questioning."

"How did that state cop miss us?"

"There was a bad accident up by Ruidoso on the other hi-way goin' north."

"What do you want to do, T?"

"Oh, let's just keep going, but this late at night there isn't very much traffic out here, so, whenever we see headlights let's try to pull off somewhere until they go by."

"Okay, you're the hot shot driver, why don't you drive us in. If we go up to Ancho and take Hi-way 55 over to Mountainair, there shouldn't be hardly any traffic and then we can drop down to 47 and hit the freeway at Belen. We'll be almost to the city."

"Sounds good to me, but I don't think my race car driving will make much difference in this rig. But, I suppose you could use a break. How come you know so much about the roads?"

"I used to be a deputy sheriff. I worked for Bernalillio County for a year before I got the job with Albuquerque PD. We backed up the Valencia county guys all the time, we had more men and they seemed to need a lot of help."

"Being a patrol officer sounds pretty simple now days, doesn't it?"

"I'll say. But I don't think I could go back. How about you?"

"I think you're right. Things have changed a lot since I worked for Del Rio's finest."

"I don't know, T, I think that what has changed is me. Sobriety seems to have made me a different person. I feel different about all of this now. I still like some parts of the job. You know, investigating and helping people, but not the danger and the lying and the deceptions that go with police work."

"Maybe you've changed, and maybe you have just set the real you free."

"Yeah, it could be. I'll see how I feel when we are out of danger, but right now, I'm thinking that this may be my last assignment."

"I don't blame you if you want out, but sobriety only made me a better cop. When I got sobered up, I could see a clear picture of what was right and what was wrong, and even the shades of gray in between. Although, I'll have to admit that this is the first time that I had to kill anybody while sober, but even with that, I think I have a good sense about when it's right to use deadly force. It is what we trained for, after all."

"I see your point, T., but those right and wrongs, and those laws that we are defending and interpreting, are man made. What worries me are the laws of God. I'm just not sure that man has the right to kill, even in the name of the law. This spiritual side of AA has really done a number on my head, I guess."

The two men drove on in silence, each in his own thoughts. Trevor was worried about the paperwork and the out come of trials and review boards while Larry was concerned with the moral implication of what he had done on this trip, and the self-recrimination he would suffer in the future. The sun was just coming up as they pulled up to the four way stop in Mountainair.

Bumper Blue was backed in next to a building where he could see the intersection. He had a greasy chicken thigh in his hand, gnawing it with much satisfaction. Finishing the thigh, he threw the bones on the dashboard where he had been throwing the bones all night. It looked like he was building some kind of a morbid alter around the plastic Jesus that the true owner had stuck there. He was dimly aware that it was lighter out side, but the booze had taken over most of the conscious part of his brain. When you are drunk, you see some things more clearly, like the silver mini-van that just turned left and started down the hill. Other things are much harder to see, like where the ignition key was and which way it turned.

Finally, he got the car started and raced the motor as he took another swig of whiskey. He didn't care if he damaged the engine or not, it was just a temporary car, anyway. He stuck the Hurst shifter into low gear and peeled out, sliding into a wide fishtail as he hit the damp black top of the early morning hi-way.

His had been a typical life story for a criminal. He had grown up in a Mississippi ghetto and after several teenage arrests, he was given the chance to enlist in the military or go to adult jail. Two years later he was issued a 'less than honorable' discharge from the United States Air Force. The last six months of his military career were spent in the brig at Kirtland AFB in Albuquerque. It seems that he gave a severe beating to the officer in charge of the motor pool where Bumper worked. The beating was a warning on an unpaid gambling debt that the Captain owed. The officer didn't see it Bumper's way and had him court-martialed. That was nineteen eighty nine. He spent the next several years mixed up in all the unsavory activities that were available to him in the south west. His best known operation was transporting everything illegal between Denver, Colorado and the Mexican Border at El Paso. He called it the 'I-25 pipeline'. Guns and drugs went north and expensive automobiles and pretty girls went south. The girls, mostly young runaways, were sold into the world wide white slavery trade. The guns and drugs kept the brothers in the cities in control of their hoods. His employees used every mode of transportation from a bicycle to an eighteen wheeler. But that son-of-a-bitch Larry Kelly had put an end to his fine fast paced lifestyle, and now it was time to pay the bill. The minivan was rounding a curve about half a mile ahead. A meaty chocolate brown hand slammed the Hurst shifter into high gear. The blue Goat lurched ahead as if the car sensed the chase coming on. Bumper's bloodshot eyes slid in and out of focus as the car tires slid around the curves with a protesting squeal.

Jackie was enjoying the ride across the Capitan Mountains, the original home of 'Smokey the Bear'. It was a beautiful New Mexico morning. Some of the aspen trees below were turning fall colors, giving the predominately pine forest a golden glow in the early sunshine. Brian Paterson's voice came through the aircraft intercom. It always startled Jackie to have someone in her ear without warning. The airships headsets were designed to emit a low "white noise' in-between transmissions to give the illusion of silence in the otherwise noisy helicopter.

"Sorry to break in on the quiet this glorious morning, but operations just informed me that they lost our patient in Ruidoso. They are going to send the body down to Las Cruses by ground transport, so we are ordered back to base. We are about four minutes out of Ruidoso. If you two want some coffee, I could go ahead and set down at the clinic for a few minutes to do a 'flight check'."

Brian Green answered first. "Naw, let's just go back. How about you Jackie."

"I vote to go back. Someone my need us and we're pretty far out on our range." She just couldn't shake the feeling of foreboding. Today, something bad was definitely rushing towards her. She couldn't visualize it yet, but it was lurking on the edge of her awareness.

The Eurocopter A-Star made a wide turn and Jackie caught a glimpse of Sierra Blanca's snow capped peak. Looking like a diamond thrust out of the forest, it was an awesome sight. She remembered her hike in the mountains a few weeks earlier and the conversations she had with Larry. She was certain that she was going to see Larry again and hoped it would be soon. The thought of a reunion with him gave her warm comfort on this morning that seemed so full of foreboding purpose. She turned her towards the morning sun, closed her eyes and let the warmth of the sunshine bath her face.

"Looks like a blue car is coming behind us, really fast. Do you know anybody with a blue GTO? You know, the hot rod car from back in the sixties?"

Larry turned and saw the Pontiac bearing down on them. "No one I know. Maybe some guy is late for the early shift somewhere."

The car was close enough for Larry to see that one large person was driving, but with both cars facing west, the early morning sunshine prevented him from seeing a face. He judged by the body size that it was probably a man.

"Looks like just one guy, do you want to let him pass?"

"We'll see. If we have to slow down too much or pull off the road and then we would be vulnerable to attack if it is someone after us."

Trevor sped up to the maximum that the road would allow and then slowed at the first straight stretch. The car behind them pulled up close and held it's position, even though there was ample time to pass.

"Well, I guess there are two choices, either this guy is a horrible driver or he has an ulterior motive."

"How far to the freeway?"

"About five or six minutes, I'd guess."

Coming out of a corner, Bumper tried to ram the left tail light on the minivan. The maneuver might have put the van through the guard rail had he connected, however, he missed and lost his element of surprise.

"Now we know, he is definitely not a friend of ours."

As a counter move by Trevor, the minivan swerved into the left lane, then back to straddle the center line. Larry had the Glock out, switched off the safety and worked the slide. The GTO hit the silver van hard, square in the back, crumpling in the van's safety bumper. Larry and Trevor both lurched forward into their shoulder belts.

"Pull over and slow down a little. Let's see if he's got the guts to face us."

When the van moved over to the left lane again, Bumper moved up on the right, but he was ready for them with his sawed off shotgun cradled across his left arm. Just as Larry caught a good look at the driver the shotgun went off blowing out the back seat window.

"Damn! It's Bumper Blue!" Larry fired a couple wild shots, more out of reaction than purpose.

"I thought you guys put him away?"

"We did. You know Bumper?"

"All the border rats know Bumper, the 'transport man'."

Now it was an all out race to the freeway. The silver minivan had no chance at out running the blue GTO, but if Trevor could keep from getting pushed over an embankment, maybe they could shoot their way out of this mess on the open ground of the freeway. Three more times Bumper was able to catch them and punch at the small van with the heavy car, and each time Trevor made the correct counter maneuver.

The two cars screamed through the small town of Belen where it was too early for any law enforcement to be on patrol. The local cop was having breakfast in the back booth of the local café and was oblivious to the speeders. The blue and silver racers left the town behind in a flash and headed for the freeway cloverleaf two miles away.

Just as the two speeding cars came into view of the freeway on ramp, a midnight blue streak crossed in front of them. It was Von Stein's MD520 helicopter. They had flown to Albuquerque, filled with fuel again and started backtracking, looking for the silver minivan.

"Looks like someone else is trying to grab our prey, boss."

"Can you take out the driver in the blue car?"

Carlos was already assembling a breakdown Browning rifle with a scope.

"Sure, just tell the pilot to hold it steady on the driver's side."

At the bottom of the on ramp the blue Pontiac caught the van hard in the right rear fender. The minivan was tossed like a flat stone onto the freeway, spinning a complete three hundred and sixty degrees as it crossed both north bound traffic lanes. An approaching eighteen wheeler was barreling down on the scene at seventy miles per hour in the fast lane. The driver had just enough time to react and swerved to the right, sliding in between the two cars. The last wheel on the trailer caught the front bumper of the GTO and spun the blue car a hundred eighty degrees. The powerful engine in the hot rod sputtered and died and it took Bumper several tries to get it started.

The motor on the van was still running and Trevor immediately took off in the direction of the truck. The truck driver had his hands full. The heavy loaded trailer would not come back into line and it was swerving dangerously from one side of the traffic lanes to the other.

Just as Bumper turned the car back to the north, Carlos completed the assembly of the sniper rifle. Bumper had the car in high gear and his foot to the floor by the time that Carlos could line up the shot. He hit Bumper in the left side of the head with a grazing shot, knocking him out instantly, but Bumpers foot was still on the accelerator. The GTO flew passed the van and exploded into the back left corner of the tractor-trailer rig. The impact was far more than the truck driver could control. The driver was experienced enough to know that applying the brakes when the trailer was swerving would jack-knife the rig, so, the eighteen wheeler was still doing over fifty miles per hour when the blue Goat hit the back end. The impact immediately unbalanced the trailer, the rig swerved in a wide arc and jack-knifed, the tractor and the trailer tipping over in slow motion.

Trevor had no time to react constructively. He stomped on the brakes and the effect was to flip the van. It rolled over twice and slid into the trailer with a dull thud, coming to rest with the passenger side down. The front windshield had blown out and Larry was trapped with his left leg caught under the dash board. Trevor hung unconscious and bleeding in his seat belt and shoulder strap. Blood was running into Larry's eyes from a gash on the side of his head and his vision was becoming blurry, a true sign of head trauma.

The blue helicopter sat down about a hundred and twenty feet from the wreck. Carlos unfolded himself from the back seat and pulled out one of his Berettas, looked around and casually walked up to the van.

"Hey amigo, you still alive?"

"Go to hell!" Larry was fighting to not pass out from the immense pain.

"We just want our property back, Señor Sully. Where are the plates?"

"Go to hell!"

"Listen if you tell me I will kill you quick, otherwise you can stay here for the buzzards."

Larry made a motion with his left arm and discovered that it was broken. Both sets of plates had been in between the seats of the van in the black backpacks. The backpacks where now draped out of the front window cavity. It wasn't his intention to give them up, but the adversary saw them anyway.

Carlos reached down and picked up both backpacks and quickly inspected them, finding the plates in tact.

"Gracias, Señor Sully. See that wasn't too hard."

Somewhere off in the distance, Larry could hear a siren. Help was coming, but it didn't look like it would be in time. The Glock was missing, or at least he couldn't see it or feel it next to him. Carlos was carrying the plates back to the 'copter, which lay just at the edge of Larry's vision. Forcing his will to overcome the pain, he pushed his arm down his right side. His goal was to reach the thirty-two caliber automatic in the ankle holster. If he stretched as far as he could, he could pull on the handle with his thumb and two fingers, but he couldn't reach the Velcro fastener. Carlos was walking back to the van, on the way he stopped and picked up the still full bottle of whiskey that had some how miraculously survived Bumper Blue's crash. Larry steeled himself and pulled as hard as he could on the small gun. The only thing that happened was that he got dizzy and weak from the pain. His head was spinning and his breaths were getting shorter. Absolutely everything hurt.

"Thank you for the plates, amigo. I also want to thank you for saving the lives of my cousins back at Al Bennette's house. They told me what you did. It's too bad I have to kill you now, but you will soon be dead anyway and it is only business."

With that Carlos took a long pull on the bottle and then poured the contents through the drivers side window, down on Trevor and Larry. It smelled delicious to Larry and nearly seduced him into giving up the fight. He shook it out of his burning eyes but his vision didn't get any better, in fact it was continually worse. Breaking free of the hopelessness of the situation for just a brief moment, Larry gave one last pull on the gun. It came loose just in time, as he was sure he knew what was coming next. Just as Carlos pulled out a book of matches, Larry thrust the gun as far out of the front of the van as he could. He didn't want to set the whiskey on fire, that was the big Mexican's plan.

Seeing the sudden movement, Carlos looked up in time to see the gun pointed at him. He had the burning book of matches in his hand, but it was too late to throw it. All that Larry could see was a big blurry shape. He pulled the trigger with all of his remaining strength and kept pulling it until all five bullets had left the barrel. Carlos fell face down on top of the matches. Larry dropped the gun, his vision was clearing and fading every few seconds. He fought to hold on, but believed he would die.

"Go to hell!" It was just a whisper, but it needed saying.

Von Stein had the plates in the MD520 and told the pilot to get going. As the aircraft started to rise, Larry saw something on the hill behind the helicopter. No it was somebody. It was Cisco! No that couldn't be. How could he be there? Cisco raised a weapon, a disposable rocket launcher. "How could that be?" Larry passed out.

The tail of the MD520 exploding into a million pieces surprised the pilot. The helicopter had not gained enough altitude to auto-rotate and slammed hard back to the ground, landing on the front shield and killing the pilot. Von Stein, in the back seat, was knocked unconscious. Cisco disappeared over the hill as the State police cruiser reached the scene.

Corporal Armondo Peña, a seventeen year veteran of the New Mexico State Police, was the first on the scene of the accident. He had just made his clear for duty call to the dispatcher after leaving his home in Los Lunas. The time was 6:58 AM, it was a clear Indian summer morning at about sixty degrees. A trucker team heading southbound had call in the accident on their wireless phone. The two drivers remained anonymous, however, they were passing by at the time when the northbound rig turned over with a blue Pontiac attached to it's rear end. The 911 dispatch center gave the call to Peña and dispatched an ambulance and a fire truck from a south Albuquerque station. Dispatch also alerted the fire and police at Belen, but their emergency people were all volunteer and the dispatch expected the Albuquerque teams to arrive first, even though the accident was just off the Belen freeway ramp.

Peña crossed over the freeway and headed south at a hundred plus miles per hour reaching the scene in just under eight minutes. The trooper pulled across a turn around just passed the overturned truck and stopped.

"My God!" He said as he crossed him self in pure Catholic fashion. He picked up the radio mic.

"423 to dispatch."

"423."

"I need lots of help out here. We have two involved cars, an overturned semi rig and an aircraft down."

"Did you say aircraft, 423? Say type."

"Affirmative dispatch. Looks like a small four place helicopter. It's hard to tell. Not much left of it. I'm sure we need a foam truck and Haz-Mat for that. Also, a couple more ambulances, officers for traffic control, three wreckers-make one of them a big one and a Lifeguard Helicopter. This looks bad dispatch. I'll be out checking for survivors. 423"

"423, be advised South Albuquerque teams are still sixteen minutes out, locals have been alerted and we have a Lifeguard helicopter in your area. The pilot advises two minutes."

"423 to dispatch, affirm, requesting dedicated frequency this incident."

"All teams for 423 incident switch to tac-22."

The necessary business took only seconds but it seemed like hours to Peña. He wanted to get into action, but protocol had to be followed for the good of all involved. As he left the patrol car, medical kit in hand, the city cop from Belen arrived. Peña assigned traffic control for him and his other officers whenever they showed up. It was time for the morning commuters to start the thirty minute drive to Albuquerque.

The truck driver was crawling down out of the truck, looking dazed and hurt.

"My partner is in the sleeper and he won't answer me!"

"Okay, we'll get to him. Are you hurt?"

"I don't know, these two crazy cars were fighting, nothing I could do. I tried, honestly, I tried."

Peña remembered his triage training. 'If they are walking and talking, move on.'

"Okay, sir. I need you to sit down over there away from the truck and remember all the details for me. Can you do that for me? I'll get back to you in a few minutes. Help is coming."

The patrolman climbed up into the truck cab. The other man laid dead, eyes staring and body at an odd angle. His guess was a broken neck. He jumped down from the truck as the Lifeguard helicopter came over the horizon from the east.

As the A-Star rotated left so that the loading doors were easier to access, Jackie took in the enormity of the situation. Her adrenaline was racing through her body as she tried to prioritize the crash scene. Finding the helicopter at a wreck with two cars and an eighteen wheeler was puzzling, so was the man lying face down in the middle of it all. Something was wrong here. It was much more than a traffic accident.

"Hey Green, listen, this doesn't feel right to me. Watch out for weapons out there, if there are survivors they may not know that what ever happened here, is finished."

"Okay, where do you want me?"

"You take the aircraft and I'll take the blue car, we'll meet in the middle at the van. We've got plenty of help coming so let's get the triage done."

The medical help jumped out of the helicopter as it touched down, each going in opposite directions. Brian quickly determined that the pilot had died in the crash and the passenger was unconscious. He carefully laid Von Stein out flat, checked for injuries and moved to the sitting truck driver as he communicated with Jackie by head set radio.

At the smashed GTO, Jackie found Bumpers heavy body impaled with the steering column. The blood loss was obviously severe. As she was checking his vitals, life and death changed places in his eyes. She moved on, joining officer Peña at the van while Green checked out Carlos.

"Tough way to start a day corporal. Did you check the semi-truck?"

"Yeah, one victim. Looks like a broken neck to me, I'm no expert, but he's definitely dead."

Jackie looked through the hole in the front of the minivan. It had the putrid smell of booze. The driver was knocked out but had a pulse. He was hanging from his seat belt, half down on the other man, making it hard to get to the victim on the bottom or to diagnose either of them. It was dangerous, but they had to be moved before much else could be done. It was Jackie's call as flight nurse and one she hated to make. A wrong move could paralyze one of these victims. She felt for a pulse on the lower man's extended arm. The pulse was weak, but he was alive covered by blood with his head back at an odd angle. She backed out of the cavity and stood up. Her mind was almost made up when she noticed the gasoline pooling by the van. One mistake and the whole scene could change to a fire or explosion.

"Pat, I need you out here. Bring a gurney, a backboard and a fire extinguisher. We've got to get these guys out quick. Do you have an up date on help?"

"South station is three minutes out, another local officer and a county deputy are here now. Belen station is rolling paramedics and a fire unit."

As Paterson brought the gurney, Jackie told Peña to see if he could enter the van through the back door. The back doors had been damaged, but Armondo was able to kick in the glass and crawl through. Jackie went back into the windshield opening and fitted neck brace to Trevor. Green and Pat tied open the drivers side door and slid the back board down behind Trevor's limp body. Jackie and Peña slowly turned him so his head and shoulders pointed at the door, being careful to keep his spine as straight as possible. It was hard work in the cramped quarters, working around the second man, Larry, only a few inches away. When they were ready, Jackie cut the seat belt and harness. After the initial weight shift, the two Brians took the weight and pulled Trevor out of the van. Peña followed him through the door while Jackie turned to the passenger.

The other man still had a pulse. Jackie repositioned herself and carefully turned the mans head. Her heart almost stopped as she realized that it was Larry. She checked his heart rate and airway, then started looking for other problems. Working her way down, he had a severe blow to the head which usually meant neck and/or back problems, however, the bleeding was from a superficial cut in the scalp. Next she notice his broken fore arm, it would be okay, no cut arteries or anything. From the position of the impact, he probably was a good candidate for internal bleeding. His stomach felt bloated and tight, not a good sign. His leg was definitely broken in several places and stuck under the crumpled dashboard.

"Larry! Oh my God! Larry, can you hear me?" No response. "We're going to get you out of here. Don't you give up on me! Larry, it's Jackie, it's Jackie and I, uh I ...." She was losing it.

"Jack are you okay over there?" Brian Paterson's calm voice was suddenly in her helmet. "What's going on, kid?"

His kind words brought her back to the professional that she was. She crawled out and stood up. The surroundings seemed surreal to her for a few seconds. Lots of help was showing up. Two ambulances, two fire trucks several police cars and the wrecker from the service station in Belen. She was in charge of this scene for the next few minutes. It was imperative that she clear her head. She took a deep breath and stomped her foot as hard as she could. She then let out the air slowly. It worked, a trick she learned from a trauma nurse who had helped train her.

"Green, report, how are the other victims?" The rest of the Double B team had the other three survivors on gurneys and were checking for injuries.

"These guys are all hurt, but nothing critical so far, Jack."

"Okay, turn them over to the ground crews and get them rolling for Albuquerque. I need you both over here this guy's in bad shape and pinned in. Corporal, get that wrecker back here, I think we need to set this van up to get him out."

She looked around. A rescue truck was just arriving.

"Dispatch, show Belen Rescue, on scene. Who's got the ball?"

Jackie waved her arm. "I do over here, I need you guys at this silver van. Do you have the 'jaws of life' with you?"

"Affirmative."

Brian Green had belted Larry to a back board, installed a neck brace and secured the back board to the seat. When they were ready, the wrecker pulled the van onto it's wheels. Eleven men helped keep the van from falling roughly to the ground. It came over and they let it down gently.

As Jackie and Green worked on stabilizing Larry, Paterson started the red and white A-Star and made ready for flight. The rescue and firemen were working as fast as they could to free Larry from the van. Nobody spoke for a few minutes. Jackie broke the silence.

"I need a time line," she said softly, her lack of emotion portraying the seriousness of the moment.

Corporal Peña answered the request. "First report was as it was happening. That was thirty-eight minutes ago."

"Pat?"

"Eleven minutes to the trauma center."

"All right, listen to me, everyone. This man has internal bleeding and we're going to be close on this one." Her voice was still calm, but authoritative. "Green get to the bird and set up for a chest drain." He looked at her blankly. "He's gonna die if we don't do it!"

"You're the boss. I've never done one."

"It's okay, I have."

Larry was free. They laid him out on the gurney and loaded him into the 'copter'. Brian handed Jackie the scalpel, tubing ready. She had cut away his shirt with scissors. Without hesitation, she used a scalpel to cut him between the ribs and inserted the tubing in the fourth intercostals space. Blood spurted threw the tube into the receptacle. Larry's chest started to subside and his breathing improved immediately.

"Go Pat!" The Lifeguard team took off for the city.

All the busy work was done until they landed. Jackie sat holding Larry's hand and praying silently.

"Is he a friend of yours, Jackie?"

"Absolutely, Brian."

"He'll make it. Thanks to you."

"Oh God, I hope so."

The helicopter touched down at 7:51 AM. Jackie turned her patient over to the trauma team and stood against the wall watching them save his life. It was an awesome feeling to have someone you love in this room. She would never forget it.

CHAPTER 17: NEW BEGINNINGS

Awareness can be elusive. Larry was aware of many people around him, for a brief time. They seemed to be busy. Then he was aware of a big discomfort, like something was invading his body through his mouth. It all faded away. And now, he was back and aware of a smell. He searched his mind trying to figure out what the smell meant. It came to him, flowers, he was smelling flowers, but he did not know what color they were. A small voice in the back of his mind said, 'open your eyes'. The voice got louder and louder until he had to respond. His eyes came open, but it wasn't a flower, it was the most kind face he had ever seen. It was Jackie and even though her face was fuzzy, Larry could see the love radiating like a bright light from her soft features. He wanted to say, 'you love me', and then he tried to say, 'I love you', but nothing would come out. He tried it again, and the word love crawled out of his dry mouth. He heard himself and the word didn't sound meaningful. The sound was more like something a hurt animal would make.

Jackie put a straw in the corner of his mouth. "Here, drink this."

Larry sucked on the straw, it felt like an awful lot of effort just to get a drink. He looked up at her and thought she was the most beautiful thing he had ever seen. A tear fell out of his left eye, making a wet spot on the pillow. Jackie smiled a warm peaceful smile.

"Hi there, do you know where you are?"

"Uni….Uni…ver…sty Hosp…ital?'

"That's very good. Do you know your name?"

"Sully, or er.. ah…Larry. My name is Larry Kelly." His voice was staring to work better now. She gave him another drink. It felt good and cool on his sore throat.

"Do you know who I am, Larry?" She was fiddling with the IV adjustments.

"Yes, you're nurse Jackie, the one I ….. Am I hurt bad?" His lips felt large and clumsy.

"Okay, that's enough, we can talk tomorrow. Go to sleep Larry and have nice dreams."

He felt sleepy, too sleepy to fight it. He tried to move his hand, to take hers, but all he could do was wiggle his fingers. "Ssss..tay."

"I'll be here." She picked up his hand and held it in both of hers as he slipped back under the blanket of sedatives.

The sun was up and the curtains were open. Trevor had a nice view of the Sandia Mountains from his bed. He hated hospitals. The worst part was that they always reminded him that he was no longer young. This morning he had to agree with the staff, he couldn't believe how much he hurt. Not the life threatening type of pain, but the dull aches that seemed to have spread to his entire body as a result of the car wreck. His ribs were bandaged, but he knew from past experience that bruised or even broken ribs must mend on their own time. The cast on his left foot didn't worry him much either. Trevor had been the recipient of many broken bones over the years. You can't ride bulls, race cars and chase bad guys for forty years without getting banged up a few times. Over the past ten years, the pain seemed to have changed. In younger years he took the pain and used it to make himself tougher. He wasn't the kind of tough guy that picked fights in bars, challenging the biggest S.O.B. in the room. No, he was the kind of tough guy who could grit his teeth and get through any situation. Pain and adrenaline shook hands in his soul. What ever it was, he could endure it, out last it, out run it, out work it or just keep going when every other man would quit. Always walking in someplace where angels would fear to go. He didn't feel like that on this morning. The re-occurring feeling was that the pain was just making him tired of it all.

Trevor didn't feel tough this morning, instead he was wondering for the first time, in a long time, about his future. Maybe he was like Larry, maybe he had changed. He understood very well what Larry was talking about when he said that sobriety had changed him. Even though Trevor had developed the rationalization mechanisms that allowed him to continue as an undercover operative after getting sober, at a deeper level, the battle went on between the things he did and the person he longed to fully become. For many years, it was just one assignment after another, always doing his job. Staying in character until he had become that character. Where was the real Trevor and what did he really want? Time will tell, but right now in this hospital bed, he just felt old. It was as if his life force had drained out on the ground next to the smashed minivan.

When the nurse came in, he was looking out the window at the hot air balloons ascending and descending as they boxed the course past his window. The colors had a happiness about them. How could anybody feel depressed watching dozens of big balloons drifting by.

"Hi cowboy, how are you today." The nurse was an attractive thirty-something woman, a bit thin for his taste but she was pleasant.

He tried to sound cheerful. "Oh, I'm good as a guy can be in my shape. Are you my new nurse, I don't remember seeing you before. And what makes you think I'm a cowboy?"

"It's your chart, the only people I know who have had as many broken bones as you have had are either cowboys or race car drivers." She laughed a little. "My name is Jackie, and I'm not really your nurse. I'm a friend of Larry's, I was hoping we could have a little talk."

Trevor needed time to think about this. "Well, about my chart, I'm both, or at least I used to be. Sixty three is a bit old for those kid games, don't you think?"

"You are only as old as you feel."

"No, I'm not that old. Today I feel about a hundred and ten." They both laughed, but it hurt his ribs and he winced.

"Do you want something for the pain? Your chart also says that you have been refusing all pain medications."

"Well, I stay away from a habit forming stuff, and aspirin might as well be sugar pills for the way I feel. Is it the annual balloon festival?" Trevor wanted to stay away from the subject of Larry until he got a better handle on who this was. Anybody could put a white uniform and pump him for information. This was his first morning where he felt in control of himself and until Captain Moffit or Larry showed up, he had to consider himself still undercover.

"Are you a friend of Bill W.'s?"

"What makes you say that?"

"Like I said, I'm a friend of Larry's, and well, you were in the wreck with him. The toxicology report said that neither of you had been drinking, but that van reeked of alcohol."

"You were there?"

"Yeah, I'm the flight nurse who picked you two guys up off the pavement. Let me tell you, it wasn't a pretty scene."

"I don't know anything about any booze in the van, but you're right, I am a member of the program. How about you?"

"Four years and trudging along, one day at a time."

"How is Larry, nobody will tell me anything? Are you, ah, Larry's girlfriend?"

It was Jackie's turn to wince. How was she suppose to answer that one. "We have a special friendship, I guess you could say that. He's still in intensive care, he woke up last night for a few minutes just after they moved him out of critical care. Listen, Trevor, is it okay to call you that? That's how they have you listed on your chart. I don't want to pry, if you are in Larry's line of work, then I don't want to ask more than I should, but as Larry's friend, could you fill me in on a few things?"

Trevor didn't feel very trusting. He hadn't been awake and in his right mind long enough to be debriefed about the operational side of things.

"I don't know, my memory is pretty shaky right now. What do you want to know?"

"As a nurse, I like to know how in the Hell you guys ended up there? Just to fill my curiosity. But, what I really want to know, is how is Larry doing, I mean, you know, in the AA department. Has he still got it together?"

"As far as I know, his sobriety is still intact, but I think he is at a crossroads. It's been a hard two or three of months for him, and me too, I might add. The wreck on the freeway, well…"

"Go ahead and tell her, you old coot." Painfully, Trevor turned his head to see Captain Moffit standing in the doorway. "The way I hear it, this little lady saved both yours and Larry's butts out there."

"Moffit, you are the sorriest excuse to pin a badge on I've ever scene. I thought they must of retired you, I've been here a couple days and you hadn't stopped by to yell at me yet."

"No need to bother a sick old man with business." Turning to the nurse, "You must be Jackie, Bob told me to say 'hi'. He'll be around later today. My name is Moffit, I'm Larry's boss and I really do want to thank you for taking care of my boys out there."

Moffit shook her hand. He was a large domineering man who carried his authority like it was a jeweled crown. Jackie patted Trevor's hand.

"Well, I'll leave you two gentlemen to talk. It was nice to meet you both, I'm going to go check on our mutual friend."

Trevor watched as she left. He liked her unassuming manner and soft ways. He understood that his friend Larry had her in his corner. Moffit had skirted the bed and pulled up a chair.

"Are you up to talking about it T.?"

"Sure Cap, if it'll take my mind off my ribs, we can talk all day."

Walking down the hallway, Jackie found herself full of anxiety. Seeing Larry in the intensive care unit was a hard thing to do. She wished that he was okay, sitting up in the room next to Trevor's. Talking and smiling, needing her, but he was not. His room was on a different floor in a different wing of University Hospital. Staff was monitoring his every heartbeat and breath. As much as she wished to see him, the seriousness of his condition took the hurry out of her steps. Larry would be in bad shape for the next few days.

Her trip through the corridors took her close to the upstairs lunch room, so she stopped for a cup of coffee. With a muffin in one hand and a large coffee in the other, she started for a table, but found herself just standing in front of the row of plate glass windows, sipping her coffee and watching the hot air balloons float by. Every year hundreds of hot air pilots converge on Albuquerque for two weeks of parties and flying. Everywhere you go, all you have to do is look up and see the graceful craft sliding by like dandelion spores in a gentle breeze. The bright colors and patterns give the sky an ever changing elegant design. Jackie thought it looked like the human race was trying to give back to God some of the beauty that he has given us.

This morning she was hoping and praying that God was on her side, or at least on Larry's side. With him laying in the bed unconscious with all the tubes and wires, she was a nervous wreck. Having slept only briefly between jags of crying and nervous fits, she had gotten up once and tried to read, but couldn't focus on the book. Another time she fixed herself a large bowl of double chocolate ice cream with Hershey's chocolate syrup on top. Finally, after a bout of nervous itching, she had drawn hot bath to try and relax. As she was use to getting up and going to work early, she was at the hospital by seven and after checking on Larry, had gone to see this Trevor guy. Jackie wasn't sure why she had gone to Trevor's room, but Larry was unable to fill in any of the missing pieces of the puzzle and she needed to know a few things. Like where he had been, and if he was still sober, and were people still trying to kill him. Any and all details were important to her at this point.

She decided against the muffin and shoved it into her uniform pocket. It was a good thing that she had decided to take a few days off from her flight nurse job. There was no way she could have worked effectively in this state. Now that Larry was back, considering the circumstances, she felt more alone than ever. Carrying the coffee, she went back into the halls. All the time she had worked here at University Hospital, she really never paid any attention to how big the hospital was. Going from ICU to Trevor's room and back was a long trip. Too much time to think. Trying to put her thoughts and emotions into perspective was almost impossible. The more she thought about everything, the more numb she became. People she knew passed her in the hall with cheerful greetings, but she didn't seem to hear them.

Finally back at ICU, she found a nurse and a Doctor in Larry's attendance. She said 'hi' and then sat quietly in the corner and let them work. The nurse changed the IV and checked his draining tubes and bandages. The doctor was evaluating the conditions of Larry's maladies. Both of them knew Jackie and neither asked why she was there. At the end of the examination the doctor turned to Jackie and reported that Larry was getting better and that after lunch they would take the drain tubes out of his chest and wake him up. The doctor and nurse left quietly. It always seemed strange to Jackie how quiet it was in ICU. She was used to the frantic noise of the ER and more recently, being on the scene with the helicopter crew where the trauma started and the noise levels were overwhelming. She spent the rest of the morning staring at Larry's sick body laying quietly in the bed. He never moved, he just lay still, breathing in and out with a bank of high tech monitors keeping track of everything except his soul. Not being able to help Larry's condition was a helpless feeling for her.

About lunch time she wandered back to the lunch room, filled another large disposable cup with coffee and headed for a table, when she spotted Suzie sitting in a corner, out of uniform and looking concerned. She wasn't in the mood for Suzie's less than mature banter, but couldn't pass her by, so she sat down with the young blonde.

191

"Hey Suzie." The need of a friend showed on Jackie's face. "This isn't your shift, what's up?"

"Good morning, Jackie. That's what I could say to you, you know. Here I am in street clothes instead of my whites, and there you are in whites instead of your flight suit."

"Yeah, well, I had some personal stuff to do and I thought I would be less conspicuous if I wore whites."

"I thought you might be here this morning. I heard that you brought in that guy Larry in bad shape. How is he? I know you had some sort of feelings for him. You know, you do have friends, and I thought you could use one now."

Jackie was truly comforted by Suzie's understanding. "Thank you. My sponsor tells me the same thing, and speak of the devil."

Katherine was headed towards their table with a tray full of lunch. When she reached the table she spread out the collection of side dishes on the table while they all passed their greetings. The oversized Indian stuck a spoon into her chicken noodle soup.

"Okay, I'm here now so we can all talk about it."

"About what?" Jackie tried to sound nonchalant and picked at the bran muffin she had retrieved from her pocket.

"You know, Larry and your feelings."

Jackie was suddenly uncomfortable. "What if I say that it's all too personal?"

"I'd just say, 'us girls got to talk about something'. If the love of my life was laying in a hospital bed, I'd want to be able to share my fears and hopes with close friends like you and Suzie, and I'd be afraid to hold it all in because that might get me drunk."

A tear rolled out of Jackie's eye, followed by another and then another. "You're right, as always. I guess I'm really scared. It's touch and go right now. You know, he has a punctured lung, a rip in his colon, a fractured skull, a broken leg and a broken arm. Just as a nurse, I would follow this case because he's so bad off, but I, ...I... I guess I love him." Jackie put down the muffin, too upset to eat. Her hands were shaking "I'm afraid that I won't have a chance to tell him how I feel."

"I'm sorry you have to go through this. I know this is hard on you, but all you can do at this point is pray for his successful recovery and take care of yourself so that you can be there for him." Katherine finished the soup and exchanged the bowl for a plate of potato salad. "And speaking of recovery, was this an alcohol related accident? I heard a rumor that the vehicle smelled like a whiskey barrel."

"No, no, the guy who was in the wreck with him said that Larry is still sober. It's amazing how fast stuff like that gets around this place. I was there and it did smell like booze, but the toxicology report came up negative on both of them."

"Wow, you've been really busy this morning!" Suzie chimed into the conversation. "Detective Jackie Grant, accident investigator."

"You talked to the other man? Who is he? What else did you find out?"

"His name is Trevor and he's in the program, too. That's about all I got this morning, he had other company. He seemed like a nice guy."

As Suzie poked holes in her empty coffee cup, Katherine was digging into her macaroni and cheese. Jackie took a deep breath to get a grip on her emotions and glanced at her watch.

"I had better get back. The doctor said that they would try to wake him up soon and I'd like to be there."

Suzie stood up and ran her fingers through her hair. "Can I tag along?"

"Sure, I guess I need the support."

"You see, now that sounds better. There's hope for you yet, Jackie."

"Well, it's not me that I'm worried about today."

"Exactly, that's why we're here. To worry about you. I've got to get back to my office as soon as I finish this cake, but Suzie can take care of you." The love shone through Katherine's sarcasm.

"Thanks, Kathy." Jackie squeezed Katherine's arm as she slipped by. The two nurses walked into the hallway.

"I appreciate you too, Suzie. You know it's hard for us alcoholics to ask for help. It never occurred to me how much I needed you girls today, but I feel a bit better now."

"You are always doing so much for me, I glad to be here for you. You know that you keep telling me that this sponsor/sponcee relationship works both ways. Remember how much you helped me when I slipped and had to find my way back. All that fear about coming back to the program on my knees and going to court over the car wreck. You got me through it all. Even when the judge gave me probation, you taught me to be grateful for the chance to face the consequences of my actions. 'Better to live in life's lessons than die in life's misery', you said. You were right, and today I really do feel grateful that I'm alive to learn those lessons. And I'm grateful to have you as a sponsor and a friend."

"Don't get mushy on me, kiddo. What ever happened to the guy whose car you wrecked?"

"He was really great in the end. Didn't press any charges and wouldn't let the insurance company go after me. He said that he was responsible for pushing me into getting drunk and high, so he had to own up to his consequences too. I offered to make payments on the smashed car, but he said cars were nothing to him. He gave me the car as a parting gift. Signed over the pink slip to me, said if it had worked out, he would have spent more than the value of the car on me, but it didn't work out so he felt he was getting out of our relationship cheap."

"He just gave you that expensive sports car?"

"The car was totaled, you know. I had to pay the towing, storage and disposal costs for it. Close to three thousand bucks."

"Even lessons come with a cash price." Jackie put her hand on the girl's shoulder and gave it a motherly squeeze.

"So tell me what happened, Cap. Did you get the bad guys? I was knocked out cold, the last thing I remember was that blue Pontiac hitting an eighteen wheeler."

"That's too bad, Trevor, we were hoping you could fill us in. We sent you guys down to Mexico to flush out Al Bennette and instead you bring us back a mess on the freeway with four unexplained deaths."

"Did you find out who all the actors were at the wreck?"

"Let's see, the black guy that died in the GTO was one Warren Lincoln Smith, you probably know him as Bumper Blue."

"The drug 'mule' guy. You say he's dead? The world will rest a bit easier over that."

"Yeah, we don't think the wreck killed him, though. Looks like he took a high powered bullet in the head just before he smashed into the truck. It is hard to tell just what the cause of death was. There was a big Mexican named Carlos something or other. Looks like Larry capped him with four out of five shots before he himself passed out. The pilot of the helicopter died on impact, but we aren't sure what brought down the bird."

"Can't help you there, Cap, I never saw a helicopter, but if Carlos was there, then that German guy must have been there, too. Did you get him?"

"Yes, we got a guy out of the 'copter with a concussion. He was mumbling in what sounded like German when they brought him into the hospital, but he hasn't made a sound since he regained his faculties. We are holding him until we can get some sort of a fix on what went down."

"You mean you don't know what you have? It worked! Larry's plan worked! That man, my dear Mr. Moffit is 'The Wolf', the biggest counterfeiter in the whole damn world! Call Interpol and be sure you have him in chains. He looked like a slippery type to me."

Captain Moffit went pale. "Just a minute here." He picked up the phone and called the police station, told them about 'The Wolf', had him placed under special guard and moved to an isolated cell. Putting down the receiver, he continued.

"Let's see, where were we, oh yeah, forensics found traces of military explosives around the helicopter. You don't know anything about that?"

"Not a clue."

Trevor reached for his pink plastic drink glass with the bendable straw in it. "So we can assume that the helicopter was the German's and that it either carried a bomb that went off or maybe it was hit by a rocket launcher or something.

Larry was shooting at Bumper with a Glock 9mm. Did they get the slug to confirm?"

"Got the slug all right, but it was bigger than a nine."

"The Mexican guy, Carlos was a body-guard for 'The Wolf', so he may have had a rifle and did in old Bumper Blue. You said four dead bodies, who else was there?"

A trucker was asleep in the back when the truck turned over. Snapped his neck like a twig. We know from his partner that they were just in the wrong place at the wrong time. We guess that Bumper was just bounty hunting for you guys or maybe trying to settle an old score with Larry. He just escaped custody a few days ago and Larry was the one who busted his operation wide open. However, most of the crooks in the great southwest were looking for you two along with the New Mexico state police, FBI and the Treasury people. I've taken care of all the authorities, there was something about a gun battle in Alamogordo? Anyway, you two are cleared on that. What I want to know is what happened to Al Bennette?"

"It's going to take some explaining and conjecture to put it all together, but we think that his man Bruno killed him during a gunfight in Chihuahua. We were there, but we didn't do it."

"You guys were in a gunfight besides the one in Alamogordo?"

"Actually Captain, a total of four gunfights and a bombing, but who's counting. I think most of the guys we killed were Italians, but we weren't the only ones shooting. It's hard to tell."

"Oh for crissakes, the paper work on this is going to take years. Dealing with Mexico is always a crisis."

"Do what you will, but I won't tell if you don't. Like I said, Larry and I didn't kill any Mexicans, they were all Italians from Chicago and probably in Mexico illegally anyhow. If Larry killed Carlos, well that was under your jurisdiction here in good old New Mexico, USA. I killed Bruno and anyone else who died in Alamogordo, so I'll take the heat there. It was in the line of duty, but Larry was going for the car when it went down."

Trevor knew that wasn't exactly true, but no need to be extradited for self-defense in the desert. The Mexican government had a history of lopsided justice.

"Trevor, you were sent on a fact finding mission that was supposed to take a couple of weeks, you guys are gone almost three months and end up with all these messes. What the hell happened down there? Did Larry blow it? You know I really didn't want him in the field so soon."

"Shit happened, Cap, you know like the T-shirt says. Larry was fine, in fact he was the best I've ever worked with. He doesn't think so, though. I think you are going to loose him, but I'll let him speak for himself when he comes around."

195

There was a long pause as both men considered what had been said. Finally Trevor added another bombshell. "Another thing, this was it for me too, I'm too old to go on like this. I'm going to take my retirement at the first of the year."

Moffit reached out and touched the older mans shoulder. "I understand old friend, you are more than due, but the border won't be the same without you keeping that ever vigilant eye on things."

The chest drain tube had been removed and the fish tank drainage apparatus had been carried off. Larry was till hooked up to the Vital Check 4400 monitoring system. The doctors had chosen to wake him up by means of his intravenous drip. The attending doctor and nurse were close by, but allowed Jackie the job of watching the patients reaction to the stimulants. It might have been a bit unprofessional, but Jackie sat on the edge of the bed with Larry's hand in hers. Nobody said anything, Jackie had earned the extra measure of professional courtesy in this hospital.

After what seemed like eternity, she felt a tightening of his hand on hers. "Come on, Larry, come back to me." More tension in the hand. "I need you Larry, come on and open your eyes." Her voice was both soft and stern, trying to create a task that his mind had to act on. She squeezed his hand firmly, held it tight for about a minute and then let it loosen.

"Damn it, Larry, I need you now!" His hand gripped hers hard and continued the hold for ten seconds.

"Open your eyes!" The eyelids fluttered open, then closed again. "That's right, come on back to me."

Larry took a fairly deep breath, as if steeling himself, squeezed her hand and opened his eyes.

"I'm here." His voice was faint and distant. Joyous tears flowed from Jackie.

"Hi there, sweet heart." The warmth of her smile seemed to bring the temperature up in the room. She gave him a sip of water with a plastic straw.

Larry tried with all his will too smile but not much was working yet. "Hi." He whispered.

Gently she touched his face. "Do you know me and where you are?"

Weakly, he turned his face and kissed her gentle hand. It gave her Goosebumps.

"Yes." Another whisper. "Thank you."

"The doctors want a crack at you, but I'll be right here." She let him go and the doctor moved in asking simple diagnostic questions that Larry could easily respond to. After a couple of minutes, the doctor gave a brief status report to Jackie and left.

"The doctor says you're going to be fine, but I'm not suppose to bother you too much."

"No bother. I want you here." He tailed off to sleep for eight or nine minutes, then he awoke with greater clarity.

"Did I drift off?"

"Yeah, a little. It's normal, don't worry about it."

"How bad am I? I'm not dreaming am I?"

"No you're here with me. Your condition is stable, they were able to fix everything. You can see you have a broken leg and arm, there were some internal things wrong, but your all fixed up now. It will just take time for you to heal. You'll be in the hospital for a while, but they will probably give us, err, you a private room tomorrow."

"Trevor, the man that was with me, did he make it?"

"Sure, he's fine, I talked to him earlier today. He said to tell you hi."

"Are you my nurse? It's so good to see you, there is a lot to say."

"I know, sweetie, I missed you too. We'll have a lot of time to talk later. No, I'm not your nurse, I'm here on my own. I'm a flight nurse full time now, I brought you in."

"I don't remember, just Cisco on the hill......"

Larry drifted off as the doctor walked back in.

"Better let him rest, Jackie. There's a pull out bed in the chair over in the corner. You should get some rest, too. We'll see if he's hungry next time he wakes up."

It was the morning of the six day after the wreck. The sun was shinning through the windows in Larry's private room. He was sore and still felt very weak. He had requested less pain medication, but he had no way to judge if the staff had made any changes. He was worried about taking too many drugs, but the nurses said he needed them to heal properly. At least he could focus a little better this morning. Jackie had been by his side throughout the past few days until last night when she went home to sleep in her own bed. Her attention towards him was more than he ever expected. She had been there to comfort him, reassure him and watch over his care. When he tried to tell her how much she meant to him, she just said they would talk about it later, but if a person could be judged by their actions, then she cared as much for him as he did for her. Somehow, amidst all this pain, her actions created a warm fuzzy spot to go to in his mind. It was better than any drugs they could give him and he knew that he would be all right.

There was a clang as a wheel chair bumped into the door frame and Larry looked over to see Trevor's smiling face being pushed through the door by an attentive Cisco.

"Jesus, you look bad partner!" Trevor's eyes where shinning with friendship. "Look what I found in the hallway." He jabbed a thumb at Cisco.

"Morning boss man." Cisco had the twinkle of mirth in his eyes that seemed to be his relaxed state.

"God it's good to see you two. Some race car driver you turned out to be. And you, I've got a question or two for you."

Cisco turned around and closed the door for privacy. "You want to know if it was really me at the wreck?"

"That's the thing that has been bothering me the last few days. I could swear that I saw you on the hill with a bazooka or RPG or what ever those things are they use to blow up stuff these days, but my vision was a little bad at the time. I think I must have passed out about then."

The Mexican, laughed and looked around in sinister fashion like they do in the movies before they tell a secret. "Okay, yous guys listen up," mocking James Cagney, "if yous repeat a word of what I's 'bout ta tell ya, we gots t'kill the lot of yas, ya here?"

Both older men laughed, both whincing in pain.

"The DEA owes fast Eddie so many favorites that he can get anything we need. We knew about the Germans helicopter, a beautiful little MD520, coming across the border. Uncle Eddie thought it was an unfair advantage, so we barrowed a DEA bird and pilot and followed them from El Paso. At the wreck, The DEA couldn't be exposed and we knew help was just minutes away so we landed behind the ridge and this LAWS rocket launcher just sort of fell out of the DEA 'copter, or at least that is what the pilot said. Well we couldn't very well let the bastard get away after all the work we put in on this case, could we?"

"You and Fast Eddie? I thought you were going to stay in Chihuahua and help Esmerelda at the Hacienda de Flores?"

"We had a little talk with Carlos and knew he was heading north. The Italians were all gone, and I got to thinking that it would be good offense to help put those guys away. No use in any of those bad guys getting ideas in the future. So, I made a few phone calls and met uncle Eddie in El Paso the day before the wreck. The rest as they say is history and all the crooks are dead or in jail. Isn't that the way these things are supposed to end? Now I can go back to Chihuahua and be a gentleman rancher."

"Sounds like some sort of Hollywood ending to me," Trevor said.

"When are you getting out T.?"

"Oh, I've already been released. They cut me loose this morning."

"What now? Are you going back to the border?"

"No, I'm going to retire in a few weeks. I feel like my cover has been compromised on the border and, you got me thinking about all this running around and shooting people, always lying to stay alive and so forth. It's time to do something with a little less pressure. I've been undercover since my wife passed away seventeen years ago. I've got a daughter somewhere in Arizona, mostly raised by her Aunt Grace. Maybe I'll look her up. What about you, still thinking of quitting?"

"It's a done deal. I haven't made any plans yet, but no more undercover cop crap for me. I won't be able to do much for a few months, so they tell me. Maybe I'll do insurance investigation or something. I don't know, like you, I've been at this way too long."

"Well, we can talk about it later, but if you want to start your own agency, I'd jump at the chance to work together."

"Thanks for the offer, I need to get well before any plans can be made, though. Working with the two of you was a great experience. If I were still a drinking man, I'd give a toast to both of you."

Cisco beamed. "I'll consider us toasted. It's been fun, but not that much fun." They all laughed. "I have to go talk to the authorities and give a couple of affidavits, then catch a jet back home, to the hacienda. The DEA just happens to have a Learjet going my way this afternoon."

Cisco shook hands and left the room. Larry and Trevor had uncomfortable silence between them. Trevor broke the spell.

"I know it's hard to get over the things we had to do, my friend. All I can say is, sometimes you are not defined by what you do, but rather who you are and what you feel about it. Don't be hard on yourself, and don't forget to forgive yourself in your prayers. We both need a heavy dose of AA right now. Have you heard from anybody in the program yet?"

Larry thought about it for a second. "Actually, there has been a whole bunch of them here all ready. Jackie, Suzie, Katherine, and some guy I barely remember named Darin that came with my sponsor Bob. Do you know any of them?"

"Not unless that's Bob the car salesman you're talking about."

"That's him."

"Yeah, we go way back to soon after I put a plug in the jug."

A candy striper brought in a lunch tray for Larry and asked if Trevor wanted one. He declined.

"Well, partner, I best roll out to a taxi and find a hotel somewhere that's a little cheaper than this one."

"Are you staying here in Albuquerque for a while?"

"Have to. This is my duty station until I retire. They say that I'm technically a US Marshal, although I don't ever remember joining the marshal service. I guess it's a catch all for us cloak and dagger types."

"Listen, Trevor, if you need a place to stay, I've got an empty house. You're welcome to it. Give me something to write on and I'll give you the address. There is a key inside the old birdhouse on the front porch. Just take it down and pull the lid off. No self respecting bird would want to live there."

"That's a fine offer, you know I think I'll just take you up on it. I'll be back to see you as soon as I can find someone to drive me. You could put Bob's number on there for me too. I could use a good sponsor right now, too."

The two ex-undercover operatives shook hands and Trevor left. Larry nibbled at his food for a few minutes, then decided to try and sleep. The thought that everything was going to be fine was very comforting. He drifted off to a peaceful sleep, in spite of the pain and physical discomfort.

Just after dinner on the tenth day of hospitalization. Jackie came into the room still wearing her flight suit. Larry had become acusstomed to her visits. She had gone back to work on the seventh day, but still spent a great deal of time in his room.

"Hi, how are you feeling this afternoon? I've got some good news for you today."

"That must be your new work outfit, it's the first time I've seen you in it."

"I'm through with my regular shift, but they are having a busy day down in the trauma center, so I'm on standby status until eight o'clock just incase they need a second helicopter crew. Like I said, I've got some news and I thought we could have a little talk, just you and me and my beeper. God willing, it will be silent." She closed the door and sat on the edge of the bed, as was her custom.

"You sound pretty serious, is this bad news?"

"Serious, yes, bad, I hope not!"

"Okay, I'm a big boy, I can handle it. Go ahead with the news of the day."

"First the good news is that the doctors seem to think you can go home. The biggest worry with your physical condition was that you would get internal infections from the rip in your colon. It seems that everything has healed well and there is no signs of infections, although they will want to monitor you for hepatitis and a few other things for several months. Your punctured lung is doing great, it will be sore for a while along with all the other stuff like where I stuck a hole in your side."

"One of the nurses told me that it was a gutsy move when you did that, but it saved my life, how could I ever thank you for something like that?"

"Just doing my job, most paramedic teams wouldn't have done that procedure, but I have several years of trauma training and I was able to stretch the rules and get away with it. Lucky for both of us."

"Well, all I can say is thank you, but that's not enough."

"You're welcome, but it's not necessary to thank me. Now there's two things I want to talk about. I'm sorry if this sounds direct and presumptuous, but it's time to talk about us. I wanted to be fair and let you heal up and get out from under the immediate effects of the trauma and surgery drugs. It would be more fair to you if I could wait even longer, but the situation dictates a certain amount of action."

"I want to talk about us, too. I've had a lot of time to think, several months actually, and the past few days, well, that's about all I could do."

"That's good, let me get this out before I loose my nerve. I want you to know a few things about me first. I've lived a single existence since I got sober these last four, almost five years. That means there has been no 'significant other' in my life. It has been hard for me to look at a man and see anything that I wanted to have in my life. It's not really the fault of the men in the world, it is really about me and how my last few years of drunkenness left me living on the street, doing awful things just to survive. I want you to know that I have a pretty spotted past. I used to go home with men just to get something to eat or a shower. I was a street whore, the next step would have been prostitution. I think it's only fair that you know what kind of person I was as a drunk. I don't want you to be surprised by anything that you might hear in the future."

"Hey there little lady," Larry's John Wayne imitation was still poor at best, "a checkered past don't bother a real cowboy none. Besides, us ex-drunks gotta stick together and forgive one another, I reckon."

"That is the point of what I'm saying here. I want us to have a future, that is if you feel like I do. I have never met anyone who has had the effect on me that you do. Oh Larry, you have been in my mind and prayers all this time we have been apart. A few times I thought I would go nuts waiting for you to come back, and the not knowing...." Her hands were trembling. Larry reached out with his good arm and took both of her hands into his one.

His voice was strong and soothing. "It's okay, take a deep breath, your feelings are safe with me."

She took a couple of deep breaths and went on, pushing back her nervousness as she pushed the hair out of her eyes. "I didn't know if you were coming back and I didn't know if you knew that.....I love you, and that love seems to get stronger all the time. It defies logic and it's uncontrollable for me. I guess, now I'm at the mercy of how you feel about me, but this feels right to me. More right than anything I've ever known." Her eyes were full of tears, her mind full of fear and her heart full of love. She had done it, committed herself to her feelings in front of the person to whom it mattered most. Every nerve in her body felt as though it would explode. The trembling turned into shaking and Larry was overwhelmed by her display of emotion.

"Jackie, calm down sweetheart. It's okay, I understand why you are so afraid and it's okay. I love you with all my heart. It is the same for me, it was torture for me to be gone for so long, but I had no choice. Some day I'll tell you about being undercover, but believe me, I longed for this day. If you have a place in your heart for a broken down cop who loves you more than life it self, then I'm your man."

"Damn, I wish I could hug you." She laid her head on his stomach and let the tears go. Larry smoothed her soft brown hair as she wept tears of joy. They stayed in that position for a long time. Long enough for the sky to turn gray with the first hint of dusk.

"I guess the only thing to find out is, your place or mine." She said finally.

"What do you mean?"

"I'm taking you out of here tomorrow morning, it's my day off, and I'm going to take care of you. So, your place or mine?"

"Do you know where I live?"

"Sure, I know lots about you. Your house is closer to the airfield where I go to work, it would be my choice."

"Well, I told Trevor he could stay there for awhile."

"That's no problem. I saw Trevor yesterday, he thinks it's a good idea, too. Your place if big enough for all of us, and besides, I work a lot so you two can keep each other company."

Jackie propped herself up and kissed Larry a long gentle kiss. It was the first time in many years that either of them had felt a loving kiss. For both of them, this was the sweetest part of a new beginning.

EPILOG

The meeting room hadn't changed much from the time that Larry first walked into AA, but after a full two years of sobriety, it was still Larry's favorite meeting place. Someone had painted a couple of walls, but that was counterbalanced by a new water stain on the ceiling. New carpeting seemed to help with the acoustics, however, there was still the sound of gentle thunder when the group stood up to hold hands and say the Lord's Prayer at the end of each meeting. Not only was the room was still here, it was still filled with the many faces of folks trudging down the sometimes sweet, sometimes rocky road to recovery. About half of those faces had been around when he had sobered up, the rest were new. Some newer than others, all were bonded by the desire to quit drinking and stay that way.

Today was a monthly 'Birthday' meeting. At the High Desert Club, on the last Friday of the month, the group had celebration for all the members who had achieved another year of sobriety during the month. Birthday cakes and cards were brought in for each of the Birthday people and each of them was expected to give a short speech about their individual experience, strength and hope as it related to alcoholism and sobriety. Some of them told serious stories, demonstrating the life and death aspect of alcoholism, others created laughter through a less than serious look at their lives and troubles.

Larry's second sobriety Birthday had been on the sixteenth of the month and he was excited about today's festivities. On the anniversary of his first year clean and sober he had been working undercover in Mexico and missed the celebration at his 'home group' here in Albuquerque. He had made a lot of new friends in the program. A look around the room was a boost to his ego. Most of the people that had reached out to him when he needed help and the ones he had helped in turn, were all here. It gave him a feeling that he was a part of something more important than any individual member. All of these friends needed each other. One of the greatest strengths of the program was the way that the hand of AA was always extended to those in need, no matter what their religion, color, sex, or social standing. Every time an alcoholic helped someone who was still suffering, it served to strengthen his own resolve not to drink.

Bob, Larry's sponsor, had told him to be very careful with his ego around his Birthday, because too much of the wrong kind of ego could set a man towards a dangerous path of self righteous pride. Larry was feeling confident about his sobriety and the hard work it had taken him to get this far. The desire to drink had been lifted from him just as the other members had told him it would be.

As the meeting was brought to order, Larry looked slowly around the room, nodding at several members who made eye contact with him. Bob, Katherine,

Suzie, and Trevor were in attendance. In a grand show of support, Fast Eddie had driven up from El Paseo. In Larry's mind, Eddie represented the past, Trevor and Bob were the present and sitting at the far end of the table, Jackie, held the keys to the future.

After the opening readings, the current Birthday people were introduced with applause for each, then the speeches started with the longest time in sobriety going first. Larry was fourth in the queue. A podium had been brought in and placed at the front of the room. As Larry took his turn behind it, his hands were trembling and it amused him to be so nervous, however it gave him a starting point for his unwritten speech.

"Hi, my name is Larry and I'm an alcoholic. I'd like to say welcome to any and all new comers and congratulations to the other Birthday people." Larry paused for a few seconds and looked at his friends with appreciation in his heart.

"First, let me say thank you to the group as a whole. You guys kept me sober, with a little help from above, and I truly appreciate it. I'm standing here trembling with nervousness because I know how important this deal is. It's about life and death, happiness and misery, freedom and bondage. There is no doubt in my mind that I would have died by now of alcoholism or it's side effects, if I hadn't been saved from this ugly disease. They told me that I was laying in my back yard, close to death from alcohol poisoning with beer and rum bottles for a bed and an unopened bag of chips as a pillow." Everyone laughed at the image, even though it was a serious subject. "I don't remember that. I do remember some guys showing up at the hospital and telling me that every thing would be better if I just listened to what they had to say. These wise men didn't lecture me on the pitfalls of drinking, they just shared there own stories in an honest way. What it was like to be a drunk, what they did to get better and how different their lives were, living in sobriety. When I got out of the hospital, I came here, to this room and you people. Here I learned a new way of life. My self esteem was restored, I learned to have faith in a power greater than myself and I learned to forgive. After a brief venture back to my old job, I realized that I was changing and becoming a different person, hopefully a better person. I could no longer function in the old life and old job I had. So, all that junk had to go to clear the way for a brighter future. Now I could tell you what that old job was, but it was classified law enforcement stuff and if I told you, then I'd have to shoot all of you." Everyone laughed again. Larry felt a wave of inner peace wash over him.

"Today I stay sober one day at a time, but I'm also building a new life. Each day of sobriety is like a brick in the construction of that new life. And I have a new tool box. This tool box comes from the 'Big Book' and from the things I learn here at meetings. I add new tools as often as I can and you people are constantly teaching me new ways to use them. A few tools that come to mind are, faith, trust, acceptance, forgiveness, willingness, honesty, gratitude, serenity, wisdom, courage, and humility. I've learned to use this process of making an inventory, confessing my defects, offering restitution to those I harm, as a way of clearing not only wreckage of the past, but also, dealing with the present. I try to be helpful to others, have faith, and stay on course." Larry paused again for a few seconds, his eyes fell on Jackie. She had her penetrating green eyes focused on his as if she was seeing into his soul.

"I guess that's about all I have to say, but I want to make an announcement to the group on a personal subject, just because you are all my friends. They say not to take on too many big things in your life during the first year or two, well, many of you know that I have started my own business as an investigator and it's doing good. For me that was down sizing, so my sponsor said it was okay." Another round of laughter. "Here is the big thing that I've waited until today to say, Jackie and I have decided to get married and you are all invited to the wedding and reception on the last Saturday of next month. Thank you for letting me share."

As Larry sat down the room was alive with clapping and congratulations. Bob brought the meeting to order for the closing. After the Lord's Prayer he invited all to stay for cake and socializing. Later, as Jackie and Larry drove home from the meeting, she interrupted the a long silence.

"You're in big trouble, mister Kelly."

"What'd I do?" He said innocently.

"You know, just wait till I get you home."

After another long silence she added, "I love you Larry Kelly."

david emm

ABOUT THE AUTHOR

David Emm grew up on an Indian reservation in Oregon, where he learned first hand about cultural diversity at the same time that he was developing a love for writing. While in school, he authored many short stories and became an editor of his high school newspaper. As an adult, much of his time was spent in the great American southwest as a businessman, and has traveled extensively as a performing musician. While working with the police in an undercover operation in Texas, he became aware of his own addiction to alcohol. Soon afterwards, he enrolled in an alcohol recovery program and has now been sober for many years. Today he operates a business in a suburb of Portland, Oregon. In this is his first novel, he hopes to combine the excitement of undercover work with the issues surrounding those who wish to stay clean and sober.

www.ingramcontent.com/pod-product-compliance
Lightning Source LLC
Chambersburg PA
CBHW030314290526
45785CB00001B/348